6

D·R·E·A·M
HEALTH

D·R·E·A·M
HEALTH

DR. BRIAN WILMOVSKY

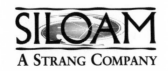

A STRANG COMPANY

Most Strang Communications/Charisma House/FrontLine/Siloam/Realms products are available at special quantity discounts for bulk purchase for sales promotions, premiums, fund-raising, and educational needs. For details, write Strang Communications/Charisma House/FrontLine/Siloam/Realms, 600 Rinehart Road, Lake Mary, Florida 32746, or telephone (407) 333-0600.

DREAM Health by Brian Wilmovsky, DC
Published by Siloam
A Strang Company
600 Rinehart Road
Lake Mary, Florida 32746
www.siloam.com

Unless otherwise noted, all Scripture quotations are from the Holy Bible, New International Version. Copyright © 1973, 1978, 1984, International Bible Society. Used by permission.

Scripture marked KJV is from the King James Version of the Bible

Cover design by John Hamilton Design
www.johnhamiltondesign.com
Interior design by Terry Clifton

Library of Congress Cataloging-in-Publication Data
Wilmovsky, Brian.
DREAM health / Brian Wilmovsky.
    p. cm.
Includes bibliographical references.
ISBN 1-59979-021-1 (hardback)
1. Diet. 2. Rest. 3. Exercise. 4. Alternative medicine. 5. Motivation (Psychology) I. Title.

RA784.W6454 2006
s613--dc22

2006021960

Neither the publisher nor the author is engaged in rendering professional advice or services to the individual reader. The ideas, procedures, and suggestions in this book are not intended as a substitute for consulting with your physician. All matters regarding your health require medical supervision. Neither the author nor the publisher shall be liable or responsible for any loss or damage allegedly arising from any information or suggestion in this book.

The recipes in this book are to be followed exactly as written. The publisher is not responsible for your specific health or allergy needs that may require medical supervision. The publisher is not responsible for any adverse reactions to the recipes contained in this book.

While the author has made every effort to provide accurate telephone numbers and Internet addresses at the time of publication, neither the publisher nor the author assumes any responsibility for errors or for changes that occur after publication.

The opinions expressed in this book are those of the author and not necessarily of the publisher, and the author takes full responsibility for errors of information. Your correspondence is welcomed. Write to DREAM Health, 1001 Cooper Pt. Rd. S.W., #140–163, Olympia, WA 98502 or call, toll free, 800-917-8368.

06 07 08 09 10 — 987654321
Printed in the United States of America

Contents

⌒

The Whole Is Greater Than the Sum of the Parts

Do you not know that your body is a temple of the Holy Spirit, who is in you, whom you have received from God? You are not your own; you were bought at a price. Therefore honor God with your body.

—1 CORINTHIANS 6:19–20

The acronym DREAM in *DREAM Health* stands for **D**iet, **R**est, **E**xercise, **A**lternative care, and **M**otivation.

I developed the DREAM Health program because every day people in pain come into my office. They are depressed, and they lack energy. They aren't happy with their lives. They may take supplements, but exercise is usually nonexistent in their lives. They suffer from many ailments. Their mental attitude is poor, and they don't take time to rest.

What they are looking for is one piece of advice, one chiropractic adjustment, or one pill that will fix everything—because what they see on TV and what they receive in many doctors' offices represents fractionalized health care that is usually dispensed only to address a short-term symptom. What they get from me instead is education, comprehensive advice, and the ability to make personal choices. My job is to tell them what they already knew instinctively—that there is no one quick fix that will furnish complete health to them. I show my patients how easy it is, with the right support, to improve their health. I tell them that optimum health is a combination of elements that add up to more energy, a healthier body, and a good mental attitude. I have learned how to help people to "flip on the switch" to the inherent healing powers in their bodies, the natural healing and protective processes with which God created them.

When my patients decide to undertake the DREAM Health program, the positive changes are dramatic. Many of them, for the first time in their lives, begin choosing to exercise, eat healthier foods, and change their undesirable habits. They find that they are aligned in body, mind, and spirit. They see that when wholeness is the goal for health instead of merely addressing pain and disease, their bodies naturally move toward health all by themselves.

I developed this program over more than fifteen years of experience as a natural health-care provider. I myself (and my family) have walked this path, lived this way of life, and found that it works. It is my great wish that you will take this information and incorporate it into your life. I want you to be able to enjoy a better state of physical, emotional, and spiritual health, too.

The focus of conventional medicine is to treat patients only after symptoms of ill health appear and conventional treatments subject you to risky drugs and invasive surgical procedures. The focus of this book is a health program that will help you care for yourself long before symptoms appear—if they ever appear at all. The DREAM Health program is proactive.

Two of the major killers of our time, cancer and heart disease, live and grow in the body for many years before any symptoms appear. Cancer generally takes seven to fifteen years to grow, and heart disease usually takes twenty to thirty years to develop in the body before symptoms sound an alarm. Historically these problems didn't have such a strong foothold in the lives of people in other cultures. That's because their way of life, which included their nutrition, their medications, and their general stress level, was different. No doubt about it, people are sicker today, in twenty-first-century United States, than they ever have been.

No matter how old you are when you begin to take care of your health in a proactive way, you will be able to forestall or even avoid diseases, even if they run in your family. If you follow the advice in this book, you will have more energy, more happiness, and more to give others. You will learn how to take care of your body, which is the temple of God's Spirit, in cooperation with the natural design with which He created it.

Come with me, and enjoy your journey to optimum health! Our passion is your potential.

—BRIAN WILMOVSKY, DC

DREAM Health: A Way of Life

⌒

The doctor of the future will give no medicine but will interest his patients in the care of the human frame, in diet, and in the cause and prevention of disease.

—THOMAS EDISON

⌒

If you came into my office for an evaluation, what would you say if I told you, "Sorry to say, my diagnosis of your problem is that you are committing slow suicide."

"What did you say? *Suicide*?"

"Yes, you're committing slow, assisted suicide. You're speeding up the aging process. At this rate, the day of your death will come much sooner than it should, and along with it, suffering from multiple lifestyle diseases and decreased cell function. As you choose how to take care of yourself, every day you're taking another step toward death. You're doing it to yourself."

Like it or not, this is my actual evaluation of your situation, unless you happen to be 102 years old already and in perfect health. The choices you make about what you eat, what kind of medical advice you seek, and how you work and rest and exercise—all of

1

these are contributing to your own early, and possibly painful, demise.

Today is the day to start making better choices. I can show you how.

GOD MADE YOUR BODY, GOD HEALS YOUR BODY

The premise upon which DREAM Health is built is that the body is endowed with its own inbuilt ability to function smoothly and heal itself when something happens to it. In essence, you are naturally well-endowed. God created you with a body, mind, and spirit, and He endowed you with the capacity to survive and thrive.

You can make decisions that support your inborn, natural, self-sustaining health—or you can interfere with it. Most of us, through ignorance, apathy, and mass advertising, do the latter.

Some of us actually seem to be making it our life goal to *sabotage* our health, and we have surrounded ourselves with like-minded folks—people who eat junk food, who prefer to watch their sports on TV instead of playing on a team, and who believe that they should always take the latest painkilling drug to eliminate their headache problems.

Instinctively, we all know that if we eat a variety of nourishing foods, our bodies will have more energy. We know that if we get enough rest, our bodies can rebuild themselves from the stresses of our waking hours, and we feel refreshed. We realize that if we live in a positive, happy environment, our whole outlook will reflect it. We know that if we get regular exercise, our bodies will thank us. And without having anyone tell us, we know that it's not so smart to ingest a substance that is toxic, even if it comes in a bottle with a prescription label.

QUICK-FIX MENTALITY

We know all of these things, but we don't listen to our own common sense. Instead, we opt for a quick-fix mentality, and unfortunately, one bad choice leads to another.

That double cheeseburger and soda you grab for lunch at the drive-through makes you feel sluggish, so you decide (again) not to stop at the gym after work. After a while, your back starts to give you trouble because you aren't in shape. Sitting at a computer all day long doesn't help. However, even though you really don't like your job, you don't feel you should take a vacation.

By now, you have gained weight, so you certainly don't want to appear at the gym anymore. Your daily stress level has stayed about the same, but somehow your ability to handle it has gotten worse. Your sleep has been affected, and you are starting to wake up stiff and sore, especially after the weekend. You are beginning to think that you are getting arthritis, like your dad, and you wonder how long you will be able to eat the high-sodium foods you crave before your doctor tells you that you have high blood pressure like your mom.

You have tried, halfheartedly, to get more exercise and go on a diet. Once you purposely took a long "mental health" weekend. But you really don't know what to do about everything. You don't even realize that you have a choice in the matter. You think these things are inevitable and that they are what everybody else experiences, too. Is that true?

Our ancestors didn't have so many choices. For better or for worse, they were often stuck with a narrow range of foods, a lot of physical hard work, few options about where they lived, and limited medical care. And yet many of them managed to make it through their whole lives without a trace of heart disease, diabetes, cancer, or any of the other diseases that are so predominate in our modern Western culture.

We have the same genetic material as they did. What has happened to us? Can we do something about our situation?

LIFE IN THE POND

Picture a spring-fed pond, surrounded by sunny green trees and filled with an assortment of turtles and fish. Birds and butterflies wing their way through the sweet-smelling air. On the far end of this pool of clear water you can glimpse the beginnings of a little stream that splashes its way through the woods, carrying the fresh water from the pond to the town in the valley.

Down in the valley, it's a different scene. The flowing water has been channeled through a succession of industries, and now it collects in another pond, this one stagnant, with no trees nearby to speak of, only clumps of discolored grass. There is a factory next to this pond, and waste chemicals have fouled the water so that it is almost opaque, with iridescent oily patches floating on the surface. Nobody takes care of this place at all. For years now, windblown roadside litter has accumulated next to the water: cigarette butts, potato chip bags, beer cartons, old plastic bags. The place reeks, especially in the summer heat.

Is it too late to restore this pond? What would you do if you owned it?

Would you take the cosmetic approach and treat the obvious symptoms of a sick environment, perhaps clean up the trash on the surface, attempt to counteract the water pollution with some special chemicals, maybe hire someone to scrape off the surface of the soil so you could hire someone else to plant grass? Or would you take a more holistic approach, halting the dumping of chemical wastes, draining out the sludge, and ending the neglect, thus allowing the pond to set itself right by the end of the summer?[1]

Like a pond, you can never be healthier than the environment you live in. But unlike a pond, you have choices about your environment. You may be living in the context of the toxic American lifestyle, but you can choose how to eat, move, think, and believe. You can continue to make good choices for as long as it takes for your body to purify itself. You can begin to enjoy the health that has been programmed into your genetic code. You can replace toxicity with purity, and deficiency with sufficiency. You can make changes in your lifestyle so that what you are putting into your body and what you are surrounding yourself with are congruent with the way God made every cell of your body. As your body replenishes itself, you can do a better job of contributing to the well-being of those around you.

Your body is able to correct a great deal of damage, even if it results from years of toxicity and neglect. Like the polluted pond, it can begin to become what it was meant to be. Your lifestyle choices do not need to remain so devastatingly different from those of your healthy ancestors, whose environments and food sources were purer than yours and who experienced much less self-induced disease as a result.

SELF-HEALING BASICS

Do you want to know how your body can purify and heal itself like the pond in my story? Do you want to understand what happens in your body when you make choices about how you take care of yourself?

Nutritional choices are prime candidates for scrutiny. Be honest with yourself: What are you putting into your mouth each day? What do you eat, drink, or swallow? Is every sip or gulp helping to build up your overall health, or are some (perhaps most) of them undermining it? We will examine nutrition in much more depth in chapter four, but for now, allow me to address you as if you had just come into my office.

Taking a look at your weight and your potential for cardiovascular disease, what I *won't* tell you is to go on a diet or stop eating chocolate. If you love chocolate, that would be the worst approach. "No chocolate" would merely be a hard-to-sustain rule to keep, a deprivation that you don't feel very motivated to maintain. You might comply for a while, but soon you would be back to supporting the candy bar industry.

I want your personal motivation to kick in, and one of the biggest helps to get you motivated will be *information*. The information I can give you will enable you to change your belief system. Once your belief system has been changed, you will naturally begin to make better nutritional choices, as well as better choices about other aspects of your life.

Ask yourself: Is this toxic to my body, or am I deficient in something? Then make choices that will provide your body with purity and sufficiency.

You will be able to put pure foods into your mouth when you become aware of the ramifications of your toxic nutritional choices. You will understand how all the rich foods, with their refined sugars and trans fats, are slowly killing you. You will begin to notice the ingredients in so many of the foods you tend to choose, ingredients such as high fructose corn syrup, which didn't even exist before 1970 but today is incorporated into 70 percent of all foods.

You will understand the chain of developments inside your body whenever you consume too much rich food. In brief, what happens is that people try to de-stress themselves with rich (toxic) food,

6

often junk food. All of the rich, toxic foods are high in sugar. So if you eat it, the additional sugar makes your glucose level spike up. (It's not just the high fructose corn syrup and refined sugar; all the carbohydrates we eat turn into sugar and push up our sugar levels.) Then your body works to create enough insulin to try to get that glucose into your cells. The more sugar you eat, the more insulin has to be secreted in order to get the energy into your cells. The more insulin pours through your bloodstream, the more your cells become resistant to insulin. And yet, as you overload your system with sugar, you will continue to pump more insulin all the time. It's a downward spiral.

In addition to understanding how the extra sugar makes your body behave, you will learn the effects of a sustained high stress level. Stress causes your body to put cortisol into your bloodstream. Cortisol is a key component of the stress response, the fight-or-flight response that is great as long as it operates only on an occasional, emergency basis. If a bear is running toward you with its jaws open, you appreciate that cortisol in your bloodstream because it lowers your insulin and shoots adrenaline throughout your system and enables you to run fast to get away from the bear.

But your body was not meant to tolerate a continuous infusion of cortisol and the chemical changes that accompany it. You were not designed by your Creator to live under chronic stress, to live in a continual state of "fight or flight." All that cortisol, remember, is lowering the effect of insulin. Here you are, already becoming resistant to insulin (which can lead to diabetes), and already you are not getting the necessary energy into your cells. Already the glucose, the sugar, is just sitting in your bloodstream, where it turns into fat (which means high cholesterol). Add to all that a lack of exercise, and you have a typical American recipe for the typical array of health problems. It's a multifaceted situation, and yet every facet involves personal choices.

So, understanding this, every time you put something into your body, you can now decide: Is this toxic to my body, or am I deficient in something? Those are the two questions you need to answer for yourself. If the cells of your body are not being bombarded with toxicity, and they are not deficient in some essential element, then they will move toward health quite naturally. Your cells were designed to be well; your body was designed to be healthy. But when we continually ingest toxins and deprive our healthy cells of their simple requirements, we are just like the sick pond above. It's all about the environment you place yourself in. Shake yourself free of the typical American mind-set (promoted by endless advertising) that it is normal to ingest toxic substances. It's not true!

> *You must replace toxicity with purity and deficiency with sufficiency.*

Are you putting tobacco smoke into your body? You are never deficient in smoke, are you? Stop and think about it.

Are you feeling tired and fatigued? Could it have something to do with those late nights in front of the TV? Quite likely, you are simply deficient in rest.

You need to replace toxicity with purity, and deficiency with sufficiency.[2] Listen to your body. Your body wants to be healthy; "health" is written into every cell of your body.

That's why you don't want to start rebuilding your health by simply depriving yourself of a sweet comfort food such as chocolate. Don't just take it away—replace it with something pure and nourishing. Add in some fresh air and some sweet sleep.

You can never be healthier than the environment you live in. Your environment includes what you eat and drink, as well as how you move, think, and believe. In order to get well, you must be immersed in an environment that is pure and sufficient for an extended period of time. You must do everything you can to expose your cells to an environment that's congruent to their function. You are not looking for a fad diet or an exercise craze; you are looking for changes in your habits. You are not trying to lose weight so you will look better in your clothing, or to gain more energy so you will be able to accomplish more. You are looking for changes that are going to move your body toward the wholeness that it was created for.

TOWARD WHOLENESS

What do I mean by "wholeness"? For that matter, what do I mean by "health"?

I often use the term *optimal health*, but I prefer to use the word *wholeism* or the phrase *holistic health*. The words *wholeism* and *holism* are pretty much interchangeable. In the context of medical care, the term includes the care of the whole person, incorporating physical, psychological, spiritual, and social factors, not simply confining medical attention to the symptoms of some disease or ailment. (The word *holistic* entered the English language after it was coined by South African statesman and author Jan C. Smuts in the early twentieth century. It comes from the Greek word *holos*, which means "whole.")

With the phrase *optimal health*, people tend to think only of physical health, or "my body." However, the phrase *holistic health* is like a word-picture for the well-being of one's whole self—body, mind, and spirit.

Standing in contrast to holism is the term *allopathy*, which considers health on a symptom-by-symptom basis. (The term *allopathy* was invented in the mid-1800s by C. F. S. Hahnemann, founder of homeopathy, to distinguish traditional medical practices from his own therapeutic approach.[3]) Allopathy is synonymous with the traditional, conventional practice of medicine as we know it in Western civilization.

9

In allopathic medicine, the most important goal is to decrease a patient's uncomfortable symptom, regardless of the effects of treatment on the patient's health as a whole. So invasive surgeries are performed and drugs are prescribed, regardless of their toxicity or side effects. The symptom may well respond, but at what cost to the patient's mind, body, and spirit?

These two health philosophies, holism and allopathy, define success as differently as they define their approaches to health. To an allopathic physician, symptom reduction is the main goal, and drugs are an accepted means to the goal. To a holistic health practitioner, those symptom-reducing drugs are considered toxic and unnatural. He prefers to use methods that enhance the inbuilt ability of the patient's own body to heal itself, even if unpleasant symptoms temporarily persist. The goal of holistic health care is to build up (or restore) the body's defenses against symptoms of illness.

It is important to understand that disease can only exist in the presence of reduced cell function. In other words, only unhealthy people get sick. If the cells of their bodies are functioning well, they don't get sick, plain and simple. My DREAM Health lifestyle is based on a vitalistic theory that says that biological forces are created, directed, and sustained by a nonmechanical, supernatural, invisible force—in other words, God. This vital force is greater than the physical and chemical forces of an organism. It directs all of the functions of a living being, and it has endowed each created being with whatever it needs to repair and sustain itself. When you get a cut, the cut will heal. If you fall ill, your body will fight the invading microorganism. When you overextend some part of your body, the resulting pain will slow you down so that you can recover.

I also use the term *dis-ease*. It was coined by Dr. D. D. Palmer, the founder of modern chiropractic care, to indicate an unhealthy, weakened state of being that is a precursor to actual diseases. When a person ingests toxins or endures physical or emotional trauma, he or she becomes susceptible to sickness. Chronic conditions can develop, and secondary ailments proliferate. But when a person works to strengthen their body in a holistic way, the state of dis-ease is transformed into a state of disease-resistance. A strong, healthy person who lives in an environment that is healthful for body, mind, and spirit does not develop dis-ease, nor does he develop diseases.

Every year for the past fifty years, the number of doctors, nurses, drugs, and hospitals has increased, not to mention the amount of money spent in North America and throughout the industrialized world on health care. Yet in every one of those years, the rate of chronic disease and sickness has increased dramatically, along with the rate of preventable death. This reveals a flaw in the system that can only be overridden by a commonsense, holistic approach to health. Good health should not be unusual. It is programmed into our genes. We need to stop interfering with God-given success and start cooperating with our Creator's original plan for lifelong health and well-being.

HEALTH SABOTAGE

The current health insurance system is set up in such a way that the majority of the coverage we receive is for the treatment, rather than the prevention of, disease. This type of health care takes us away from the innate healing power that we all have inside and puts that power in the hands of others, often with disastrous results.

Many people grow sicker and die every year from conventional, allopathic medical care because their poor bodies have become so weakened by lack of preventive health care. They suffer from ongoing stress, poor diets, lack of exercise and rest, and no spiritual life to speak of.

Add to this the potentially harmful effects of conventional medical care itself. A recent study of 37 million patient records reveals that an average of 195,000 Americans died due to potentially preventable, in-hospital medical errors.[4] This study exposes almost twice as many deaths from medical errors as were reported in the 1999 Institute of Medicine report, "To Err is Human," and it tallies the cost of these preventable deaths at more than $6 billion annually. Regarding the results of the latest study, Dr. Samantha Collier, vice president of medical affairs at HealthGrades, a health-care quality company, said, "If the Center for Disease Control's annual list of leading causes of death included medical errors, it would show up as number six, ahead of diabetes, pneumonia, Alzheimer's disease and renal disease."[5]

Milton Silverman, MD, former professor of pharmacology at the University of California, has been quoted as saying, "Our figures show approximately four and one-half million hospital admissions annually due to the adverse reactions to drugs. Further, the average hospital patient has as much as thirty percent chance, depending how long he is in, of doubling his stay due to adverse drug reactions."[6]

The bottom line is that sickness is extremely profitable for the health-care system of the United States. Paul Zane Pilzer, economist, presidential advisor, college professor, and author of the book *The Wellness Revolution,* states that "approximately one-seventh of the U.S. economy, about $1.5 trillion, is devoted to what is erroneously called the 'health-care' business. Health care is a misnomer, as this one-seventh of the economy is really devoted to the sickness business—defined in the dictionary as 'ill health, illness, a disordered, weakened, or unsound condition, or a specific disease.'"[7] Pilzer also characterizes "the sickness business as *reactive.* Despite its enormous size, people become customers only when they are stricken by and react to a specific condition or ailment. The wellness business is *proactive.* People *voluntarily* become customers—to feel healthier, to reduce the effects of aging, and to avoid becoming customers of the sickness business. Everyone wants to be a customer of this earlier-stage approach to health."[8]

This is what I am talking about, and it is my passion: introducing people to the wide world of preventive care and wellness. I like to use what I call the "fireman analogy." It goes like this: If your house is on fire, whom will you call? The fire department, of course. They are going to come and use all the means at their disposal to put out that fire—water hoses and axes and ladders. They will chop down your door and break your windows and put holes in your walls and spray down the roof and the contents of your house in their all-out effort to quench every trace of flame and smoke. If you're lucky, they will save the life of your house.

But after the fire is out, your house is in terrible, terrible condition. So whom do you call then? Not the fire department again, surely. Who can repair the damage and bring the house back to a normal, healthy state? You will call reconstruction specialists and maintenance specialists, won't you? They are analogous to the natural health-care doctors, as the firemen are analogous to the conventional medical doctor.

What's happened in our society, however, is that we use the firemen not only to put out our fires but also to rebuild our bodies. It doesn't work very well. What is meant for an emergency (which may be due to neglect in the first place) doesn't provide suitable care for reestablishing strength, health, and wholeness.[9]

Common medical practices are designed to detect illness (sound the fire alarm) and treat symptoms (bring in the fire trucks). The medical industry is highly qualified to do this. But they are not designed for fire prevention. Doctors are trained in how to treat the symptoms of an illness, but nobody consults them for advice about preventing illness in the first place.

Of course, by the time the symptoms of an illness have become detectable, the illness has already been growing in a person's body for years. Think, for instance, of arterial sclerosis, heart arrhythmias and other irregularities, cancers, diabetes, diverticular disease, emphysema, fibroid tumors, hypertension, osteoarthritis, internal polyps, renal failure, tuberculosis, and even tooth decay. Preventive care works to stop the formation of the illness in the first place. How much better it would be to focus our energies on the holistic promotion of good health rather than having to deal with the recovery of lost health and the repercussions of emotional and physical pain that occur with treatment of full-blown illnesses.

CHANGING YOUR MIND

Until we change our way of thinking about our health, individually and collectively, we will continue to experience poor health and high medical costs.

But if enough people begin to change their way of thinking, not only will their health improve, but also the price of health care can come down. In the future, ideally, people will carry high-deductible health insurance for catastrophic events only, while their employers fund "wellness accounts" for as little as $100 or $200 a month, which will provide employees with $1,200 to $2,400 a year to be spent on health club memberships, nutritional products, wellness education, and alternative care. This would dramatically reduce medical costs while improving people's health even more dramatically by promoting prevention.

It is a matter of changing your mind about the fundamentals of how to achieve good health. Instead of following a piecemeal way of living, one where you try to achieve health by looking for the next pill, exercise, or type of care that will fix everything, you want to start taking a holistic approach. The key to whole health is to treat the whole person. When the whole person is better nourished, better rested, better strengthened through exercise, and more sensibly treated by medical professionals, the person's healthier body can eliminate diseases and problems that may have persisted for years. Medical intervention becomes a rare event. Optimal health can be achieved—and maintained—to the point that it becomes the norm. I often quote Dr. James Chestnut on this basic tenet of wholeness care: "Health is normal, and normal is optimal."

We need to retrain our thinking. We need to trust that the God who created us has equipped our bodies with the power they need to do the work of healing. Instead of living in fear that when the outside forces of ill health "get you," your options are limited to other outside forces such as drugs or conventional medical treatments, you need to trust that you can cooperate with your body as it regenerates itself toward optimum health.

I call the people who come into my office my "practice members," not my "patients." Practice members are people who want to be there, who take personal responsibility for being proactive in their health care. It's like joining a health club. By becoming a practice member, they are taking an active step toward becoming better parents, spouses, employees, employers, doctors, lawyers, construction workers, computer programmers, engineers, schoolteachers, or whatever they are.

"Health is normal, and normal is optimal."

They start by realizing how the twenty-first-century American lifestyle has sneaked up on them and has made them sick. My practice members know that when they run, their cardiovascular strength improves. When they push forcefully against their muscles, their muscle strength improves. When they adopt good posture (even for sleeping), all of their systems work more smoothly, and they feel stronger. When they eat proper nutrients, their bodies can use them as building blocks for stronger, healthier bodies and minds. When they get good rest and adequate relaxation, their connection to God is improved and enhanced, not to mention their connection to the people around them. When their mental outlook is consistently positive (not full of fear or disbelief), they can achieve much more, and they can continue to improve their level of health. They know that their immune systems will become stronger, which means that their bodies can do what they were designed to do—keep healing themselves every single day. The whole person becomes healthy and strong.

This can be *you,* and it can start today. Even at a distance, you can become a "practice member." There are no guarantees in life, but I believe there is one guarantee that I can make: your body will function better and be stronger and healthier if you adopt the DREAM Health lifestyle.

LOOKING BACK

Health is a matter of choices. If you adopt a new attitude about taking care of yourself, and if you remain motivated to make good choices every day about your diet, your rest, your exercise, and your alternative care, you will be able to enjoy a happier, healthier, more abundant life.

By making positive choices to improve your health, you are, of necessity, steering clear of your old choices, which have had the negative effect of added toxicity to your life. From now on, you will be making choices with an eye to supplying sufficiency for your deficiencies and purities for your toxicities. Sufficiency or deficiency? Purity or toxicity? You can choose. DREAM Health will show you how. It's a matter of life or death.

Unplugging From the Matrix

⌒

Do not conform any longer to the pattern of this world.

—ROMANS 12:2

⌒

In *The Matrix*, moviegoers watched the dramatic plot unfold—artificial intelligence machines had taken over the world as we know it. Human beings had been plugged into a computer version of twentieth-century life, and they didn't realize that the *real* reality was different, because they lived in a "pod," with their minds connected to and manipulated by a computer program. Gradually, the main character started to understand that his reality was not what it seemed. He began to realize that there was part of life that he had never known about, and he began to persuade others to believe him.

In twenty-first-century America, it is as if we are plugged into a matrix-like reality that is not what it seems—the matrix in our case is an unexamined reality regarding how we view our health. Without recognizing what's going on, essentially we accept the worldview of traditional medicine, a worldview in which the only way to find health is through drugs or surgery. We don't recognize the more comprehensive view, in which "health" means a balanced combination of body, mind, and spirit, a reality in which crises that require drugs or surgery are the exception rather than the rule.

LEADING CAUSES OF DEATH

In our twenty-first-century American health matrix, the death statistics alone are telling.

Every year, the leading cause of death in the United States is heart disease, which kills between 675,000 and 700,000 people annually. The second-ranking cause of death is cancer, which takes more than 500,000 lives each year.[1] Alarmingly, although there is no system in place by which the numbers can be tracked with exactness, the medical care methods and drugs prescribed by the medical profession end up causing as many annual deaths as the diseases for which they are prescribed to cure. The authors of the paper "Death by Medicine," released in 2003 by the Nutrition Institute of America, say that 783,936 Americans died the prior year from a combination of adverse drug reactions, medical errors, infections and bedsores, malnutrition, and unnecessary procedures.[2] According to an article for the Knight-Ridder news service, "It is estimated that U.S. drug fatalities run 100,000 a year. There is no way of confirming the numbers because there is no reliable way to track and investigate problems with drugs. Doctors are not even required to report bad drug interactions."[3] These mortalities cut across racial lines and include Americans in all age groups from all parts of the country. We need to wake up and recognize that putting our welfare into the hands of the medical system is risky business!

Carrying on with our poor lifestyles, we wait for our bodies to wear out from heart disease and cancer; then we seek medical care via toxic drugs and invasive surgeries, which can be just as deadly. How crazy is that? Who got us to think like that? The current medical system, which includes good, well-meaning physicians, but which is a setup for mistakes. Logically, whenever drugs or surgeries are employed, there is plenty of opportunity for human error and adverse reactions.

ADVERTISED TO DEATH

If you turn on your television set at almost any hour of the day or night, chances are that you will see an advertisement or some type of broadcast about prescription drugs. We are bombarded with information about new drugs on the market that will treat a wide variety of ailments, while at the same time we hear that antibiotics and other drugs are losing their effectiveness against infection and illness.

No matter what your problem is, even if it's something that your grandma could have cured with a cup of chamomile tea, the ads will tell you the latest pill to take or the best type of surgery that will fix it. Are you troubled with insomnia? Perhaps you should try a sleep aid such as Ambien. Don't blame the advertiser if you wake up in the emergency room after "sleep-driving" by mistake:

> Reports about patients who eat, cook and even drive in their sleep after taking Ambien have raised questions about the safety of the insomnia drug and have led some to criticize the nation's growing use of prescription sleep aids.... With doctors writing 26 million prescriptions for Ambien a year, even rare events could affect a lot of patients, says Michel Cramer-Bornemann, a doctor at the Minnesota Regional Sleep Disorders Center in Minneapolis.
>
> Recent research paints a picture of disturbing behavior. Ambien is one of the top 20 drugs found in the blood of drivers pulled over by Wisconsin police, says Laura Liddicoat, a supervisor of the forensic toxicology program at the Wisconsin State Laboratory of Hygiene.[4]

Now, I believe that the responsibility is on each of us to know what we are putting into our bodies and what the potential side effects might be. But because of the explosion of drug advertising in recent years, consumers demand to try new drugs, and doctors can be too easily pressured by their patients to write more frequent pre-scriptions for more popular drugs. The patient may feel that this is the best way to "take control of my own health," but it can be dangerous. We have been advertised into a quick-fix mentality. While patients may be better informed than ever about disease and medicines, they may be taking unseen risks when they rely on what they hear in drug advertisements. They may believe, for instance, that every advertised drug has been approved by the United States Food and Drug Administration and that therefore it has been clinically tested and proven safe. This is not true!

The responsibility is on each of us to know what we are putting into our bodies and what the potential side effects might be.

According to Katharine Greider, author of *The Big Fix: How the Pharmaceutical Industry Rips Off American Consumers,* drug makers "increasingly insist on designing studies and controlling the raw data; some investigators may not even be allowed to see all the numbers. If results are unfavorable, drug makers are sometimes able to prevent them from coming to light."[5]

Brian W. Vaszily, editor and columnist for Illinois-based Mercola.com, writes, "Sadly, these days all 'FDA-approved' really means is that a drug is approved to reap even more ridiculously high profits for its manufacturer."[6]

SIDE EFFECTS OF SIDE EFFECTS

In any given day, you will come into contact with at least one person (it may even be you) who is taking at least one drug—whether it is ibuprofen, antibiotics, or heart medication. Quite aside from misdiagnosed and mismanaged treatments, the side effects alone can create a whole new set of problems. Even the side effects have side effects.

Take the drug Vioxx, for example. It was prescribed for pain. And yet before it was taken off the market in 2004, the FDA estimates that it may have contributed to 27,785 heart attacks and sudden cardiac deaths between 1999 and 2003. This is a staggering number. When patients come to me (for pain, for instance), the situation becomes very personal to me, because if I don't properly educate them about adopting a lifestyle of wholeness, they could end up being one of the next Vioxx statistics.

I counsel many patients who are suffering from some kind of negative side effect from taking drugs. These patients say they are fed up with taking drugs that make them feel worse rather than better. They tell me that they are "sick and tired of popping pills."

Just think about it. What drugs are designed to do is to make biochemical changes in your body. In the effort to quell unpleasant symptoms, your cell functions are disrupted.

Take the antibiotic amoxicillin, for instance, which is widely prescribed for many different types of infections. The U.S. National Library of Medicine and the National Institutes of Health list the following potential side effects from amoxicillin: upset stomach, diarrhea, vomiting, skin rash, itching, hives, difficulty breathing or swallowing, wheezing, or vaginal infection.[7] You or one of your children may have experienced some of these side effects.

The effects of a single drug may be bad enough, but most people don't stop there. If you are an older adult or you know someone who is, you know that the average older patient takes several drugs at the same time. Sometimes a drug is prescribed to correct the side effects of the first, and so on. The drugs affect your body, and they affect each other. And we call this "health"?

We should not consider it normal even for the elderly to be on constant medication. Instead, taking our cue from past cultures (which lacked today's meds, and they didn't suffer the same disease rates we do today), we should look at how we can change our environment to make it a healthier one.

ANTIBIOTICS

The news reports that are the most telling are about drugs that are losing their effectiveness over illness. Let's look at one of the most frequently prescribed class of drugs—antibiotics. Over the years of over-prescription of antibiotics, many patients have not finished their full course of treatment; some of the bacteria were killed off, but the bacteria that were left behind have begun to develop resistance to the drugs. As other people encounter the new, modified "superbugs," the drugs are no longer effective for them, which puts everyone at risk.[8] Along with this, our healthy bacteria (probiotics) are also killed off; our healthy bacteria are an essential part of our immune and digestive system.

The World Health Organization reports that up to half of all pneumonia and meningitis cases are now resistant to penicillin. In some countries, 98 percent of gonorrhea cases are resistant to penicillin. Up to 60 percent of hospital infections are caused by drug-resistant microbes. In fact, 14,000 patients die in the United States every year from drug-resistant bacteria picked up in hospitals.[9]

Cipro, an antibiotic that is used against many infections, including inhalation anthrax, "is becoming increasingly ineffective against other dangerous germs because of overuse, a study found....Many germs [have] grown resistant to fluoroquinolones, a class of antibiotics that includes ciprofloxacin, known by the brand name Cipro."[10]

According to the World Health Organization, "Existing drugs are gradually becoming ineffective as antimicrobial resistance spreads. We have seen simple antibiotics for simple infections become unusable. This forces us to resort to much more expensive antibiotics with many more side effects. We face a situation of great urgency."[11] The following statistics are summarized in the WHO publication *World Medicines Situation*:

- Worldwide, it is estimated that half of all medicines are inappropriately prescribed, dispensed, or sold, and that half of all patients fail to take their medicine properly.

- An estimated two-thirds of global antibiotic sales occur without any prescription, and studies in Indonesia, Pakistan, and India show that over 70 percent of patients were prescribed antibiotics. The great majority—up to 90 percent—of injections are estimated to be unnecessary.

- The inappropriate use of medicines is not only widespread, but it is also costly and extremely harmful both to the individual and the population as a whole. Adverse drug events rank among the top 10 causes of death in the United States and are estimated to cost that country between $30 and $130 billion each year.

- Growing resistance to antimicrobial medicines is a particularly serious challenge in countries at all economic levels and results largely from inappropriate prescribing and use. For the treatment of malaria, chloroquine resistance is now established in eighty-one of the ninety-two countries in which the disease is endemic.[12]

Pharmaceutical companies are finding it difficult to develop new antibiotics and other drugs fast enough to replace those that have become ineffective, although they are doing the only thing they know to do—looking for more potent drugs—while really losing the race.

The over-prescription problem is a real one, but physicians are not the only ones to blame for the over-prescription of antibiotics. The farming industry routinely gives antibiotics to cattle, pigs, and poultry to keep them free of symptoms of disease and to promote growth. Some people fear that as we eat these animals, we are ingesting the antibiotics that they have taken. Even if this is not the case, antibiotics that are over-prescribed for animals are losing their effectiveness to fend off infections just as they are for human beings. Overuse of prescription antibiotics is producing strains of bacteria that are simply resistant to any type of antibiotic treatment.

HARM FROM BIG PHARMAS

Why do traditional medical doctors prescribe so many drugs? The whole premise of the medical community is in treating symptoms rather than underlying causes. Medical personnel are schooled by pharmaceutical companies to dispense drugs on a regular basis in the treatment of symptoms of disease. Because so many young boys are on Ritalin today, social critics such as author Greg Critser are calling our kids "Generation Rx."[13] This is not OK!

Pharmaceutical companies make it attractive for doctors to not only prescribe medicines but also sometimes to prescribe the most expensive ones on the market. Drug company representatives are doing their job well. A large percentage of doctors see pharmaceutical sales representatives almost monthly and receive gifts from drug companies every year. Simple logic would lead to the conclusion that the more money a drug company has to spend on gifts and trips to doctors' offices, the more often doctors on the receiving end of this would prescribe their particular drug. The doctor's choice of prescription may have nothing at all to do with what is in the patient's best interest. It may simply be economics at its finest. Paul Pilzer wrote, "In the United States, doctors typically prescribe completely different treatments for the same ailment depending on which drug company has the dominant market share in their region."[14] Doctors often learn about new drugs and treatments from sales representatives of drug companies.

Meantime, as I have already mentioned, funding for impartial research studies is hard to come by, because so many studies are funded by vested interests. Much of the time those who provide research funds have a direct financial interest in the drug or the topic under evaluation. An article in the *British Medical Journal* reports that "finding senior medical researchers or clinicians without financial ties to pharmaceutical companies has become exceedingly difficult." Furthermore, the author writes, "There is a brewing conflict between the world's leading medical campuses and big pharmaceutical companies. Twisted together like the snake and the staff, doctors and drug companies have become entangled in a web of interactions as controversial as they are ubiquitous."[15]

> Discussing studies from around the world the article revealed that 80–95 percent of doctors regularly listen to drug company representatives' advice and information on drugs, "despite evidence that their information is overly positive and prescribing habits are less appropriate as a result." The article revealed that doctors receive multiple gifts from drug companies every year, and that medical doctors tend to deny the influence this might have on their judgment.... "Many professional societies rely heavily on industry sponsorship, just as their medical journals rely on drug company funded trials, company advertisements, company

purchased reprints, and company-sponsored supplements, despite the consequent conflicts of interest and evidence that sponsored supplements are more promotional than other articles."[16]

Is it logical to rely on the traditional medical community to give you health advice if their sources of information are motivated more by financial gain than by wellness? The answer is a clear *no*.

Fueled by economic concerns that are becoming increasingly more important to many doctors than the needs of the patient, the traditional medical structure is due for a collapse. Before it's too late, we must unplug ourselves from the matrix of traditional medicine and look at the logic of the system. Once we make the decision to take the power back, to rely on our natural God-given self-healing ability, there will be no going back to the traditional medical community.

LOOKING BACK

My passion about taking that power back begins with you understanding the half-truths and outright lies you have been hearing for so many years. Don't let traditional medicine scare you into thinking that your health and wellness can only be controlled by forces outside of yourself, in the form of drugs. This is simply not true. It is my belief that you must take drugs only when absolutely necessary (not for every quick fix), or you will never experience optimum health. Once you understand this one principle, you are well on your way to the path of DREAM Health.

How to Handle Stress

Attitude...is more important than facts. It is more important than the past, than education, than money, than circumstances, than failures, than successes, than what other people think or say or do. I am convinced that life is 10 percent what happens to me and 90 percent how I react to it.

—CHARLES SWINDOLL

Stress—"The Epidemic of the Eighties"—that's what *TIME* magazine called it in 1983. (You can see their uptight, maxed-out, stressed-out cover guy on the Web site of the American Institute of Stress.[1]) Here we are, more than twenty years later, and Americans (as well as people from many other developed countries) are even more uptight, maxed-out, stressed-out, and anxious. You would think we would have conquered stress the way we have conquered polio. Far from it. We are still conducting studies about it and writing about it, the whole time stressing out some more.

On top of that, we are still coming up with new and improved "stressors" with which to crowd our busy lives: Internet access in every home; computer and video games; pagers and beepers; ever-improving cell phones and personal digital assistants. We are overwhelmed with choices: which TV channel to select, which DVD to watch, which convenient, up-to-the-minute service to order. Even our automobiles come equipped with more features than we can learn how to use.

So we seek balance. It is possible to find it. That's what this chapter is about. *Balance* is a key word in the DREAM Health program.

IDENTIFYING THE PROBLEM

Stress consists of physical, emotional, and chemical factors. It creates tension that is felt in a person's body or in the emotions or both. Physical stress can come from illnesses, injuries, surgical procedures, or the strain of vigorous or prolonged physical activity. Physical stress can also come from the opposite—enforced, sedentary inactivity. Chemical stress is a form of physical stress. Chemical stress includes substances such as alcohol, tobacco, and drugs (everything from aspirin to chemotherapy). Emotional stress occurs when a situation seems unmanageably difficult, and it can include relational issues, financial problems, and grief over the loss of a loved one.[2]

Not surprisingly, all stress factors are interrelated. Physical tension results in emotional tension, and vice versa. Chemical toxins create physical and emotional reactions.

While I think we all understand that stress is a common part of everyday life, it is important to understand that some stress is actually a by-product of how we *perceive* a particular situation. Each person relates differently to different situations. For example, a couple I know are complete opposites in one regard—the husband absolutely detests completing paperwork, especially filling out forms, while his wife finds it stress-*relieving* to do the same tasks. Completing such detailed tasks stresses out the husband. His wife, on the other hand, enjoys the process, and she knows she will feel even better when the paperwork is completed and the details are out of the way. Thankfully, these two individuals balance each other nicely, because, of course, she takes care of the paperwork, which she finds relaxing, and he handles other tasks that she finds stressful. The stress factor is all in the individual perception of the situation.

We can't always find someone else on whom to offload our stressful tasks, can we? So how do many of us handle that uncomfortable, stressed-out feeling? Dr. Scott Hannen portrays the common default method of dealing with stress:

> Looking for ways to escape the stress of the day, [many people] sit up late at night watching TV or surfing the Internet, losing the hours of rest they need to replenish the body's energies. Even the kind of entertainment many people choose stresses the body. The programming they watch involves violence, terror, murder, bloodshed, loud noises, screams, shrieks, collisions and trauma. People are receiving these mental impulses on a regular basis without realizing that the body interprets all of it as stress.[3]

Sound familiar?

Here we are, surrounded daily with demanding stimuli, and we decide to relieve the strain with what? More stimuli. Our bodies are doing the best they can to respond to everything. They are trying to protect themselves from the ongoing barrage of stressors: physical, emotional, spiritual, environmental, chemical, circumstantial, relational, financial, and much more.

There's a catchall term for the way our human bodies try to protect themselves from all of this—*allostatis*.[4] It comes from the Greek root words *allo* and *stasis*, which mean "variable" and "stability." Your body's allostatic response to the stress load is to readjust itself continually in an effort to achieve the balance of stability. This is a good response, and it helps you survive and thrive. However, we all know that you can have too much of a good thing. A good response to stress becomes an overused response, which leads to an increasing number of bad results in your body, mind, and spirit.

The stress load itself is called the "allostatic load." From the point of view of body health, a high allostatic load incurs a high cumulative cost. In other words, although I probably don't need to tell you, too much stress is bad for your health! When your body, mind, and spirit are not allowed to escape the load of stress, eventually something breaks down. You get sick. You develop aches and pains. You get clumsy or crabby or depressed. The stress affects every cell of your body, which breaks down their function and leads to disease.

> *Learn to relax. Your body is precious, as it houses your mind and spirit. Inner peace begins with a relaxed body.*
>
> —NORMAN VINCENT PEALE

You may be able to get along for a time without any alarming symptoms, but in the long run your body and brain are like a rubber band that has been overstretched too many times. What happens? You develop "functional symptoms and syndromes, decreased cognitive function...abdominal obesity, [and] increased risk for hypertension and cardiovascular disease, insulin-dependent diabetes and decreased immune responses."[5]

READY FOR ACTION

Our bodies were never designed to live in an environment that initiates a state of chronic stress. You've heard of the "fight-or-flight" response, when a threatening situation arises, and your body reacts by releasing chemicals, specifically cortisol and adrenaline, which make you instantly able to confront or flee the danger.

Cortisol and adrenaline are steroid hormones made in your adrenal glands that regulate blood pressure, cardiovascular function, and your body's use of proteins, carbohydrates, and fats. When these hormones are secreted into the body, they trigger physical responses. Your blood sugar level rises, additional red blood cells are released to carry extra oxygen, your blood vessels constrict, your pulse quickens, your blood pressure rises, and your digestion comes to a halt. These hormones also cause a breakdown of muscle protein, which releases amino acids into your bloodstream. (The liver uses these amino acids to produce glucose for energy, which allows your body to have the focus and energy it needs for the stress at hand.)

Now, if the danger is a real one, this is exactly the right response. If you are driving down the highway and suddenly there is an accident, the fight-or-flight response will make you able to perform feats you never could do under ordinary circumstances. It may save your life. But when your system is flooded routinely with abnormally high levels of stress hormones, they become hazardous to your health. Your blood pressure remains elevated; you suffer from insomnia; you become chronically fatigued, depressed, and moody; your libido declines; and your high blood sugar levels may precipitate diabetes. Your immune system is weakened, your blood cholesterol count rises, your heart is strained, and your cognitive function is compromised. Over time, your body starts to deposit more fat around your waist, which increases your risk for heart disease, cancer, and other illnesses.

Cortisol, which regulates your waking and sleeping cycles, is normally more abundant in the morning so that you can wake up and get to work. It's supposed to be lowest at night so that you can go to sleep. When you are under chronic stress, the daily cycle is disrupted. What happens? You have insomnia. Then, lacking adequate sleep, you are more likely to fall prey to infections and diseases, which you will not be able to recover from quickly because your immune system is compromised. You may notice problems with digestion and elimination, because the stomach acid hastens the digestive process and stimulates the colon. In addition, you may feel hungrier and you may overeat, especially at night.

IT'S EVERYWHERE

Stressors occur in every aspect of life, but more research has been conducted about on-the-job stress than any other kind. The National Institute for Occupational Safety and Health reports that:

- Twenty-five percent of workers view their jobs as the number one source of stress in their lives.

- Seventy-five percent of employees believe that they have more on-the-job stress than did employees a generation ago.

- Twenty-nine to 40 percent of workers feel "quite a bit" or "extreme" stress at work, or they report their job is "very or extremely stressful."

- Twenty-six percent of workers said they were "often or very often burned out or stressed by their work."[6]

Other studies conclude that up to 80 percent of workers feel stress on the job, with nearly half of them saying that they need help in learning how to manage stress and 42 percent saying that their co-workers need such help. Ten percent are concerned about an individual at work they fear could become violent, 9 percent are aware of an assault or violent act in their workplace, and 18 percent themselves experienced some sort of threat or verbal intimidation in the previous year. Fourteen percent have felt like striking a co-worker. One quarter of the workers surveyed said they have felt like screaming or shouting because of job stress, and more than 25 percent have yelled at fellow workers. Fourteen percent said they work where machinery or equipment has been damaged because of workplace rage.[7] After a workday surrounded by stressed-out colleagues, up to 62 percent of workers routinely find that they end the day with work-related neck pain, stinging and tired eyes, sore hands, and trouble getting to sleep at night.[8]

Recent surveys have concluded that an estimated 95 million Americans suffer a stress-related problem every single week. As much as 80 percent of all illness is stress-related, and 85 percent of all industrial accidents are linked to personal worker behavior that includes signs of stress.[9]

These are alarming statistics! And besides the human toll, on-the-job stress results in huge costs to employers in the form of absenteeism, accidents, diminished productivity, employee turnover, medical and insurance costs, and workers' compensation awards.

Of course, some people actually prefer staying at their place of work, because it's less stressful there than going home at the end of the day, where much emotional stress awaits them from their spouses and children and family problems.

The fact of the matter is that whether it's at work or at school or at home, today's high level of aggravation, worry, and stress-producing circumstances exacts a big toll on everyone.

DO YOU HAVE TOO MUCH STRESS?

Early signals of stress overload are easy to miss. You may come home from a hard day at work to a relatively calm and happy family scene, only to keep feeling just as stressed out as you did during the day. Logically, your situation does not demand anything like the fight-or-flight response. But your body is beginning to be trained by prolonged exposure to threatening circumstances to pump out cortisol and adrenaline. You feel agitated and irritated.

The signs and symptoms of stress vary greatly from one person to the next, and it is therefore imperative that each of us learns to identify the ways in which we experience stress personally—the warning signs that are specific to us—and learn to take steps to better manage our overload. If your allostatic load increases (in other words, if you keep on being stressed out), you will notice some of the signs and symptoms of stress overload listed in the charts.

PHYSICAL SIGNS AND SYMPTOMS OF STRESS

- Increased, "pounding" heart rate
- Elevated blood pressure
- Sweaty palms or cold hands
- Headache
- Diarrhea or constipation
- Muscle twitches
- Itchiness
- Changes in eating habits
- Nausea
- Insomnia and sleep disturbances, resulting in fatigue
- Repeated colds and illnesses
- Muscle aches
- Hair loss
- High or low blood sugar
- Lack of coordination
- Lower back pain

EMOTIONAL SIGNS AND SYMPTOMS OF STRESS

- Feelings of helplessness and dependency
- Poor emotional control
- Excessive moodiness
- Withdrawal from responsibility
- Irritability

- Angry outbursts
- Hostility
- Depression
- Restlessness
- Difficulty being flexible or adapting to changing circumstances
- Anxiousness
- Diminished initiative
- Feelings of unreality
- Feelings of over-alertness
- Constant worrying
- Diminished personal involvement with others
- Lack of interest in life
- Tendency to cry
- Tendency to be critical of others
- Impatience
- Narrowed focus
- Reduced self-esteem

COGNITIVE-FUNCTION SIGNS AND SYMPTOMS OF STRESS

- Forgetfulness
- Blurred vision
- Errors in judging distance
- Reduced creativity
- Loss of sense of humor
- Inability to make decisions
- Lack of concentration
- Diminished productivity
- Lack of attention to detail
- Decreased reaction time and coordination

- Disorganization of thought
- Lack of control or need for too much control

BEHAVIORAL SIGNS AND SYMPTOMS OF STRESS

- Increased smoking
- Increased alcohol or drug use
- Overeating
- Social withdrawal and isolation
- Listlessness, accident-proneness
- Aggressive behaviors
- Compulsive behaviors
- Procrastination and indecision
- Workplace absenteeism or tardiness due to stress-related illnesses

REDUCING THE LOAD

My goal is to help you decrease your allostatic load. Besides identifying the signs and symptoms of an already-existing stress overload, each of us needs to become aware of our *threshold for stress.* Understanding early signs can help us intervene and manage our stress reactions before they get out of control. John Newman, author of the now-classic book *How to Stay Cool, Calm and Collected When the Pressure's On,* identifies the five phases of stress:

1. Gearing up. The initial energizing reaction gears you up for action. You're excited. Your muscles are charged, your perception acute. All systems are go.
2. Peak performance. You channel that energy. You are

focused on your goal and you make things happen. You have a positive, high feeling. You are intense.

3. Using up. If you remain in high gear, your mind starts to wander, your muscles tighten, and you can feel the strain on your system. You're tired. Your ability to communicate well dwindles, as does your energy supply. Illness may set in at this point.

4. Running down. If you continue operating under constant stress with no breaks, no time for recuperating, then your physical and mental states continue to deteriorate. You may have impaired judgment and more severe stomach, bowel, or cardiovascular problems. Chemical dependence and inappropriate behaviors are common. Chronic fatigue may also begin.

5. Exhaustion or burnout. Your energy reserves move toward depletion. You feel totally exhausted, mentally and physically. You become disillusioned; you devalue yourself and your spirit collapses. Severe depression is not uncommon.[10]

WHAT CAN YOU DO ABOUT STRESS?

If you've read this far, you've already taken the first steps toward lessening your stress. You've learned what stress is and how it can affect your body, and you've learned some early warning signs.

The ability to recognize when you are exhibiting some of the first stages of a stress response is crucial to arresting the stress cycle at the earliest possible moment. You want to stop the negative effects of stress before they do damage to your body.

Just as we as individuals react differently to stress, each of us has our own unique way of beginning a stress cycle. I call these "stress markers." My own stress marker is when my family starts to comment that I am irritable or unapproachable. For others, it might be developing back pain or a sense of anxious agitation. You must find out what your particular stress markers are in order to recognize the pattern and intervene.

A good way to get help in identifying those markers is to ask your friends and family, who will no doubt be able to tell you what they have noticed about you. Your stress triggers and early stress markers will be different from theirs, but they will have learned what to watch out for as they relate to you.

Don't throw out the baby with the bathwater.

Remember the key word: *balance.* In your effort to thwart unhealthy stress cycles, you don't want to alleviate all of the stress in your life. After all, a certain level of stress, or stimulation, is needed for optimum performance. If you have too little stress, you won't be able to motivate yourself to do anything. You can become lethargic, bored, and dissatisfied with life. Too little stress can be just as bad as too much stress.

All of us do our best work while under a certain amount of stress or stimulation. We need to be engaged in what we are doing, alert, and "with it." Stress management specialist Audrey Pihulyk writes:

> Stress can be compared to the strings of a violin. When the tension of a string is too loose, it vibrates slowly producing a low pitch sound. When the tension is too tight it vibrates too fast, giving a high screechy sound. If the string is tightened beyond a certain point, it will break. However, when the string is adjusted just right it produces beautiful and harmonious music. Likewise, too much stress in our lives can be disastrous and too little stress can be a negative force. However, just the right amount of stress can be a positive force enabling us to work at peak performance.[11]

Researchers from the University of Kentucky and the University of British Columbia, Dr. Suzanne Segerstrom and Dr. Gregory Miller, evaluated almost three hundred scientific papers on stress and posted the results of their survey in the *Psychological Bulletin* journal. The papers covered studies of some nineteen thousand individuals in North America, and they note the dynamic tension between "good stress" and "bad stress," especially in terms of the immune system:

> They found that a short burst of stress, such as that caused by giving a speech, may strengthen the body's immune system by triggering the immune system–boosting "fight or flight" instinct that dates back to when early man was threatened by predators.
>
> But long-term stress such as an injury or trauma that caused permanent or life-changing damage, such as having a long-term disability, losing a partner or spouse or being abused as a child, appeared to wear out the immune system, leaving people more prone to infections....
>
> "Stressors with the temporal parameters of the fight-or-flight situations faced by humans' evolutionary ancestors elicited potentially beneficial changes in the immune system," the researchers said. "The more a stressor deviated from those parameters by becoming more chronic, however, the more components of the immune system were affected in a potentially detrimental way."[12]

In other words, when your situation is one that requires a burst of energy and a sharp mind, your body's stress response is a gift, and you can be grateful for it. This is a healthy kind of stress response. Your stress response does not become unhealthy until your life becomes so full of fight-or-flight situations that it makes you break down physically and emotionally.

The important thing is to become aware of how your own body, mind, and emotions function. If you've had a stressful day, simply recognize that reality and find a way to "dial down." You don't have to *be* the stress, and you don't have to keep it. Just becoming aware of it as such will calm down a lot of your mental gymnastics.

WIN-WIN APPROACH TO STRESS

To help yourself achieve the healthy balance that you want, I recommend that you grow in your understanding about yourself. Then you will be better able to choose a course of action that will work for you. What can you do to reduce your allostatic load? How can you learn to better allow stress to roll off your back?

"You cannot run from stress," says Dr. Redford Williams, who teaches psychiatry and behavioral sciences at Duke University. "You cannot hide. You need evaluation tools so you can make a rational decision about chilling out or coming out swinging to change the situation."[13] Redford and Virginia Williams, in their book *In Control: No More Snapping at Your Family, Sulking at Work, Steaming in the Grocery Line, Seething in Meetings, Stuffing Your Frustration,* recommend that you first take stock of your immediate situation, and then that you take their "I AM Worth It" approach to arriving at a solution. "I AM Worth It" is an easy-to-remember acronym.

- **I...** The *I* of "**I AM** Worth It" stands for: Is what's stressing me out *Important*? Or is it simply a minor annoyance?

- **A...** The *A* of "**I AM** Worth It" stands for: Is my response to the stressor *Appropriate*? Am I responding the way any other person would, or am I overreacting?

- **M...** The *M* of "**I AM** Worth It" stands for: Is the situation *Modifiable*? Can it be changed?

"Worth it"

Last, you ask yourself to examine what's at stake in taking some action. Is it *worth it*? For example, the Williamses say, "Will it help or hurt you to go over your new manager's head to discuss your overwhelming workload, or would it be more prudent to wait until your new boss has settled into the job?"[14]

The most critical aspect to distinguish is whether your stress-producing situation is a valid one and whether it's possible to fix. If the problem is too minor to dwell on (such as coping with bad traffic on your commute) or beyond your control (such as the weather), your best choice might be to take a moment of calming meditation upon God's Word.

Keep things in perspective. Sometimes the words we use to describe our stressful situations are emotionally charged and can worsen the way we feel. "My workload is *killing* me" or "My kids are driving me crazy" are overdramatic statements. Or you may think, *My life is always like this*, or *I'll never understand this*, which are statements that lock you into a limited perspective.

Watch out for all-or-nothing statements. Your subconscious mind accepts them as true. When you catch yourself making one, change it to reflect reality: "My workload is really making it tough right now," or "Sometimes I don't understand this." When you say to yourself, "She is always mean to me," your subconscious will never give you the option of seeing that person any differently. Ask yourself a question, "Is that 100 percent true?" Hardly anyone would be mean to you 100 percent of the time. Now you can modify and qualify your statement to better reflect reality.

You can also employ some self-talk, repeating a statement to yourself that helps to relieve the pressure, such as: "One day I'll laugh about this." "This is a learning experience." "This is just one more chapter for my book."

A sense of humor and a positive attitude are guaranteed stress-reducers. If you avoid taking things too seriously, you can focus on the positive side, and you're already on the way to finding a solution to your situation.

In general, you might also want to consider how to modify your diet or exercise plan so that you will be healthier and more resilient. In her news report titled "Keys to Managing On-the-Job Stress," Heather Cabot said, "Physical activity, including walking, swimming, running and even gardening for at least 30 minutes, three times a week can elevate your mood and help you cope."[15]

LOOKING BACK

I believe that while the Industrial Revolution and the "Information Age" have allowed us to be far more productive than ever before, they have increased our stress load dramatically. I believe that the next revolution will be the wholeness revolution—we will learn to regain our natural balance and heal ourselves.

The only way to produce a DREAM Health lifestyle is to decrease the stress load on your body. You can identify and reduce the outside sources of stress, and you can improve your body's ability to adapt to inevitable stressors.

However, it is never a good option to take medicines to alleviate stress. Instead, learn more about the components of a balanced, health-promoting lifestyle, and make them a part of your life. You're not shopping around for the latest fad diet or quick fix. You are making changes that are congruent with the way you were designed to live. You are making healthy changes that will last a lifetime—and that will make your lifetime a lot more fulfilling.

Diet: Keys to a Balanced Approach

⌒

And the LORD God made all kinds of trees grow out of the ground—
trees that were pleasing to the eye and good for food.

—GENESIS 2:9

⌒

As Americans, we are used to taking our food for granted. We have more than enough of it. We don't have famines, and even occasional shortages are more of an inconvenience than a crisis.

Ironically, however, our high standard of living seems to equate to a poor state of health. As our food has gotten easier and cheaper to obtain, its contribution to our overall health has decreased significantly. An estimated 65 percent of adults in the United States are either overweight or obese, and as much as 30 percent of all adults over the age of twenty are defined as obese, with these percentages rising annually.[1] People complain that they are stressed-out, over-busy, depressed, and anxious. Their lifestyle, which includes fast food eaten on the run, washed down with caffeinated and sugared beverages, makes them fatigued, overweight, and blind to their self-perpetuating predicament.

This chapter is a wake-up call for Americans who want to take their health into their own hands. You *can* take hold of the reins of the runaway horse called Nutrition, and I want to show you how. Too many nutrition resources are little more than fad diets. They contradict each other and vie for our attention, making it nearly impossible for us to figure out the truth. In the following pages (along with Appendix A), you will find an overview of nutrition that is sensible and balanced.

With this information, you can make changes that will greatly improve the quality of your life—and extend your lifespan for many more health-filled years. As you begin to change over to a new way of thinking about nutrition, you will notice benefits right away.

OUR NUTRITIONAL HERITAGE

Two hundred years ago, our ancestors enjoyed whole vegetables, fruits, grains, and meats that were indigenous to the area of the country in which they lived. They may have had much more limited selection than we do today (what Connecticut housewife had heard of an avocado in 1800?), but the food they ate tended to come from the fields, forests, farms, lakes, and oceans nearby. Some of it came from their own well-tended gardens and chicken yards.

In those days, the soils were not yet stripped and depleted by overfarming and modern agricultural methods. They weren't yet polluted by pesticides and herbicides. So the food that came from the earth, whether it was in the form of plant or plant-fed animal, contained a wealth of vitamins and minerals and other nutrients. Add daily outdoor exercise into the mix, and you have a good recipe for a balanced, healthy lifestyle.

Today, the vegetables and fruits that we harvest and eat have been inundated with toxic additives to make them grow fast, stay "fresh," and stand up well to being shipped across the country to your supermarket. If you want to buy a local vegetable in season, you often can't even find it in your local supermarket, because its line of supply stretches to another state.

Today our meat and fish are stuffed full of the equivalent of fast food so that they can be brought to market quickly and at the heaviest weight possible. When a beef cow has been stuffed with a cornmeal diet in the feedlot, the resulting meat is marbleized with tenderizing fat (the glucose from the cornmeal is converted to saturated fat), but that fat contains an increased amount of highly saturated palmitic acid, which is bad for the health of the person who consumes the meat. Our ancestors ate grass-fed beef, which is lower in saturated fat, full of essential vitamins, and provides more omega-3 fatty acids because of the grass on which the animal has grazed. (Other foods provide a more plentiful source of these healthy fats, but why trade them for saturated fat?) These days, even when cattle start off as grass-fed, they are taken off grass when they are shipped to the feedlot to be fattened for market, whereupon they immediately begin to lose the omega-3 fatty acids that they have stored in their tissues.

Today, even if you find a way to obtain food that is pesticide-, insecticide-, herbicide-, and hormone-free, the nutrient quality of the soil has continued to erode steadily as crops are harvested over and over again, which compromises the resulting nutrients in the food you buy. Intelligent supplementation has become a necessity for a healthy lifestyle.

Our ancestors ate naturally fed animals, birds, and fish. By and large, their meats were leaner. They consumed much less refined flour and processed cereals, and far fewer dairy products. Their fruits and vegetables were grown in better soil. Their preparation methods were less complex (i.e., more pure), and they could not have conceived of today's vast number of fast-food restaurants, fad-driven recipe books, and televised cooking programs.

Our ancestors' genetic code was the same as ours. (Our genes have not been "refined" along with our flour and sugar.) So we cannot blame our genes—no matter what you may hear tomorrow about the latest "gene for cancer"—for our ill health. We can, however, blame our food-raising and consuming practices. In my opinion, the medical establishment and the pharmaceutical companies are trying to convince society that disease is a genetic problem. Clearly, it is first and foremost a *lifestyle* problem.

I am on the bandwagon for diet reform. I believe that we need a revolution in the way we think about our nutrition. I will even go so far as to make this statement: "If it has a label on it, it's *not* food." How many ingredients does it take to make a crisp green pepper or a crunchy walnut? Along with avoiding pesticides, herbicides, antibiotics in animal feed, and a host of other toxic substances, we need to draw the line at all "empty calories" to which we have grown accustomed. We need to adjust our eating habits to include more live food and a healthier daily eating schedule. Read on to find out more about how to make *good* nutritional choices for yourself and your family.

TAKING AIM AT THE AMERICAN DIET

The emergence of the fast-food industry has created a significant difference in how we think about our food intake. A hundred years ago, most people ate at home, and they ate food that they had grown at home. Today there is a fast-food restaurant on almost every corner. We obtain our food from these establishments almost as often as we eat at home.

Our lives seem to be so fast-paced and stressful that too many of us simply lack the time and inclination to prepare our food at home. We hurry through the drive-through and grab breakfast, lunch, and dinner, and our children grow accustomed to the taste. And, as we know all too well, the cheap, processed foods served at these establishments are largely composed of what are called "empty calories"—white flour, excess fat and sugar, little or no nutrients.

The nutritional breakdown of a traditional burger and fries dinner, even without "super-sizing," can contain 1,250 calories, 65 grams of fat, 1,650 grams of sodium, and 9 grams of sugar.[2] This typical drive-thru repast uses 100 percent of the typical person's daily-recommended allowance of fat grams, and 69 percent of the recommended grams of sodium. This doesn't include a drink or any dessert items!

In order to compete with fast-food restaurants, the food industry has accommodated our need for fast, quick, and tasty foods in the supermarkets, lunchrooms, and convenience stores. These "foods" are downright toxic because of their empty calories and the preservatives they contain to increase their shelf life. From my point of view, preservatives are well named, because they will simply preserve you in your unhealthy lifestyle.

"If it has a label on it, it's not food."

The ingredients in packaged dinners will not supply your body with the necessary fuel, vitamins, and minerals to keep you healthy. Consequently, after you have eaten one of those meals, your body will continue to cry out for fuel—so you will eat more food and gain weight. Your unhealthy eating leads to a host of problems that can be traced to your toxic lifestyle, from heart disease, cancer, and diabetes to cognitive disorders, bowel and bladder difficulties, and overall sluggishness. We are slowly polluting ourselves to death.

It is becoming painfully clear, even if you put fast food and its equivalents aside, that the Western diet is high in saturated fats, trans fats, and refined sugars and flours. All of these foods lead to increased acidity in our blood, which tilts our pH balance in the wrong direction. The normal bacteria that live in our intestinal tracts cannot thrive in an acidic environment. Our ancestors' diets promoted a more alkaline environment, where their natural pro-bacteria could flourish and provide health protection. They didn't have to take Zantac or Prilosec to decrease their stomach acidity. They didn't have to worry about taking supplements or choosing foods that contained probiotics to replenish what had been lost.[3]

Acidity and alkalinity are expressed on the pH scale, which ranges from 0 (very acidic) to 14 (alkaline, or "basic"). Normal blood is slightly basic, with a pH that is slightly above the halfway point (7.35 to 7.45). If a person's blood has a low pH, it is acidic, which cre-ates a hospitable environment in the body for yeast, fungus, and unhealthy bacteria. Add to that the overuse of chlorinated water and antibiotics, which kill off the normal, helpful bacteria that we have left, and you have our current situation. The only way to tilt the balance back in the right direction is to eliminate the culprits in our diets, replacing the toxicity with purity.

Fortunately, filtered water and fresh, enzyme-rich produce and meats are available, and although they may not be as convenient and inexpensive to obtain and prepare as a quick pass through the nearest McDonald's, the positive effects of making them a staple of our diets can be truly remarkable. I believe that, in the long run, this kind of food will be a lot cheaper for your health.

GOOD FOOD BASICS

The three main energy sources for your body are carbohydrates, fats, and proteins. A deficiency in any of the three areas can increase your risk for chronic diseases. It's not so much a question of ratios of carbohydrates, fats, and proteins as it is a question of the quality of the sources of those energy sources. My recommendations for daily food intake, in brief, are that you obtain 40–65 percent of your fuel from carbohydrates (preferably in the form of fruits and vegetables), 30–40 percent of your fuel from fat (from organic meats and fish, vegetables, nuts, and select oils), and 20–30 percent of your energy from protein (from lean meats, fish, eggs, and vegetable sources). In combination with calorie-producing energy sources, you need water, water, and more water.

Here is a short food primer for you:

Carbohydrates

Carbohydrates are the primary source of fuel for your body; they provide energy to your cells. Your body seeks to burn carbohydrates first, before it burns anything else for energy.

The two categories of carbohydrates, simple and complex, are converted to glucose in your body, which is what your body uses for fuel.

Simple carbohydrates. I refer to simple carbohydrates as "rocket fuel" because they consist of refined white sugar products—table sugar, candy, cake, syrups, sweetened cereal—as well as refined starches such as pasta. These foods burn fast and hot in your body, and they provide few, if any, vitamins and minerals. Foods that are high in sugar often have a high amount of fat as well, and they tend to be high in calories. They can fill your stomach and satisfy your cravings to the point that you stop feeling hungry for more nutritious foods. They can cause rapid changes in your blood sugar levels, which can make you feel tired. If you eat large amounts of simple carbohydrates over a period of years, your diet can lead to diabetes and hypoglycemia (low blood sugar) due to insulin resistance. (As a matter of fact, insulin resistance due to toxicity from both diet and stress combined with dietary deficiencies is the backdrop of almost all chronic diseases.) Even if you eat them in moderate amounts, simple carbohydrates don't allow your body to function optimally, which sets the stage for a weaker body overall. Your weaker body will more readily fall prey to diseases, injuries, and other forms of debilitation.

Complex carbohydrates consist of fruits, vegetables, and whole grains. I refer to these as "high-leaded fuel." These foods burn at a slower rate and provide your body with more sustained energy. Complex carbohydrates provide energy *and* vitamins, minerals, and fiber, all essential components of your optimal health.

In general, for obvious reasons, complex carbohydrates such as whole-grain products, beans, fruits, and vegetables are better for you than simple carbohydrates such as desserts and soft drinks. Complex carbohydrates assist in your digestive process by giving you fiber and helpful bacteria, and can help to decrease your risk of heart disease. Besides, the nutrients in fruits and vegetables are more easily absorbed by your body, and they contain antioxidants that help reduce health risks such as cancer.

In general, it is best for you to consume complex carbohydrates in the morning, because they stimulate your body to start metabolizing fuel, which sets your metabolic rate higher for the rest of the day.

A carbohydrate deficiency can be signaled by decreased secretions from your mouth, nose, and eyes; muscle weakness; and an inability to concentrate.

Fats

Fats are the second most valuable fuel source for your body. They possess the valuable functions of transporting and helping with the absorption of fat-soluble vitamins, cushioning your body's organs, and maintaining your body temperature. Dietary fat is found in most animal foods such as meat and milk, in oils, and in most processed foods. Extra dietary fat is converted to body fat and stored in fat cells, which can then be used later for energy.

However, fat is not burned as a fuel source until the body has utilized any and all carbohydrates that you have eaten recently. At that point, your body initiates a process called *ketosis,* which is a natural adjustment to your lack of new carbohydrate energy sources. Ketosis shifts your body into gear to derive energy from your stored fat. Both carbohydrates and fats are broken down into glucose to provide fuel for your body. However, the process of ketosis requires both glucose and oxygen in order to operate. If the glucose has not been provided by carbohydrate consumption, your body will start breaking down muscle and organ tissue first to obtain it. This is why an extreme, non-carbohydrate diet may not be a good idea.

Fat gets a bad rap. Your body *needs* fat in order to function well, although you should be aware of which fats are better for you. "Bad" fats, for example, are found in meats, junk foods, margarines, and dairy products. These fats are saturated fats, and they will solidify at room temperature. "Good" fats (commonly called essential fatty acids, with omega-3 fatty acids at the top of the list) must be ingested each day because your body cannot manufacture them. They contain DHA (docosahexaenoic acid) and EPA (eicosapentaenoic acid), which help to ensure that your nervous system and organs function properly and smoothly. Omega-3 fatty acids are found in flaxseed oil, canola oil, green leafy vegetables, vegetables, salmon, tuna, trout, and sardines.

You must understand that a high intake of cereals and grains increases your intake of omega-6 fatty acids, which can then outweigh the benefits of omega-3 fatty acids in your diet. The diets of most Americans are heavy on the omega-6 fatty acids and light on the omega-3 acids, especially the diets of children, whose diets often include almost no omega-3 fatty acids. The neural networks inside a child's brain develop slowly, and development can be defective if a child lacks omega-3 fatty acids. Some researchers have traced connections between omega-3 deficiency and ADHD as well as other forms of brain dysfunction such as depression and anxiety.

Protein

Your body is composed primarily of water and protein. Your bones, muscles, skin, hair, and internal organs consist of protein, as do your enzymes, which influence every function of your body. Your immune system requires a constant supply of protein in order to build new cells. Good sources of protein include meat, fish, eggs, cheese, beans, lentils, nuts, and seeds.

You need to eat foods containing proteins every day. Your body obtains most of its energy from carbohydrates and fats, but it dips into your protein stores for energy if necessary. You should eat enough protein so that your body doesn't have to deplete the proteins from your liver and muscle tissues.

My recommendation is to eat a high-protein diet when you are trying to change your metabolism and insulin resistance. If it is more convenient for you, you could combine your protein consumption with leafy vegetables (not with starchy vegetables such as potatoes or yams). Some people advocate eating your veggies first and then your meat, or vice versa, but no studies have been done to prove the benefits of either approach. Surely our early ancestors ate as their circumstances dictated—either all vegetable, or all meat (after successful hunting), or a combination.

Symptoms of protein deficiency include the following: increased secretions from the mouth, nose, and eyes; cold and swollen hands or feet; muscle cramps; low tolerance for exercise; and bleeding gums.

Water

Water comprises a very high percentage of body weight—up to 70 percent in a lean, adult male. Everyone has a slightly different percentage, depending on their age, gender, and relative proportion of fat. For this reason, water is the most important part of your diet. All of your body systems depend upon it. Water flushes out toxins and carries nutrients to your hungry cells. Water cushions your spine and your joints and protects them from deterioration.

I don't recommend tap water, which can carry too high a proportion of contaminants and chlorine (added to kill harmful bacteria). I prefer to drink distilled water with some lemon or lime juice added for the sake of maintaining my body's pH balance. I also recommend that people drink water purified by a reverse-osmosis filter. The quality of the water in your home and workplace will help you decide what kind of filtration or purification system to use.

How much water should you drink? As the hours of the day and night pass, water disappears quickly from your body. You lose some with every breath you take, as well as through your sweat and urine. Therefore, to maintain healthy function, you need to replace the lost water during your waking hours. Many people fail to consume enough fluids, with resulting ill effects such as headaches, fatigue, and muddled thinking. They

HEALTH TIP:

Consider keeping one 16-ounce water bottle at home, one at work, and another in your car. Being surrounded with easily accessible water will remind you to drink even if you are not feeling thirsty.

don't realize that they need to drink more, because they don't feel thirsty. But the feeling of thirst is a late indicator of the need for more water. We should keep hydrated despite the absence of thirst. In general, if your fluid intake makes you produce one or two liters of colorless or slightly yellow urine a day, most likely it is adequate.

Along with many advisors, I recommend that you try to take in at least 64 ounces (the equivalent of eight 8-ounce glasses) of water every day. However, all of your water intake does not need to be in the form of plain water. A report from the Institute of Medicine states, "About 80 percent of people's total water intake comes from drinking water and beverages...and the other 20 percent is derived from food."[4] The same report quotes Lawrence Appel, professor of medicine, epidemiology, and international health at Johns Hopkins University: "While drinking water is a frequent choice for hydration, people also get water from juice, milk, coffee, tea, soda, fruits, vegetables, and other foods and beverages as well."[5] If you increase your intake of fruits and vegetables, most of which have high water content, you will help your body stay hydrated. Cucumbers, for example, are nearly 100 percent water, by weight. Avoid sugary drinks and frozen desserts; you can meet all of your body's requirements for water without compromising good nutrition.

The bottom line: water is good for you! Besides, it's calorie-free, fat-free, easily available, and inexpensive.

A word about fiber

In an effort to eat healthy, people often drink nutritious beverages to the excessive exclusion of consuming foods that need to be chewed. This is a mistake. Whole foods are vital to our diet because they provide fiber. Without fiber, our digestion, energy absorption, and elimination are compromised. Many people assume that fiber means whole-grain products, but many other whole foods, especially whole vegetables and fruit, supply natural fiber. If you put a thin sliver of broccoli or apple under a microscope, you can see clearly the beneficial fibrous cellular structure that helps to bulk up your food intake.

Fiber supports the natural bacteria that populate your intestinal tract, and it keeps the food moving through your system. Yes, eating a lot of vegetables and beans does increase flatulence (gas). The intestinal bloating comes from the fermentation of the fiber by your healthy intestinal flora. This is entirely normal. Don't avoid fiber-containing whole foods because of it. Simply experiment until you find a level of fiber that you can live with, and enjoy the increased health benefits of your improved diet. Fresh fruits and vegetables are better sources of fiber than grains.

EATING ORGANIC, EATING PURE

All of my nutritional advice is firmly based on the assumption that the best foods are straight from living sources (rooted in the ground or walking, flying, or swimming) and that they are untainted with additives of any kind.

Earlier in this chapter, I mentioned the steadily depleting condition of the nutrients in the soil in which America's food is grown. This is an unquestioned fact of our present-day existence. Most food-growers compensate by using artificial fertilizers to make their worn-out fields more productive, and they also use toxic pesticides, herbicides, and insecticides in an effort to protect their susceptible food-producing plants from threats.

The meat and fish industries do the same thing. Take the cattle industry, for example. According to John Robbins, natural health expert:

> Traditionally, all beef was grass-fed beef, but in the United States today what is commercially available is almost all feedlot beef. The reason? It's faster, and so much more profitable. Seventy-five years ago, steers were 4 or 5 years old at slaughter. Today, they are 14 or 16 months. You can't take a beef calf from a birth weight of 80 pounds to 1,200 pounds in a little more than a year on grass. It takes enormous quantities of corn, protein supplements, antibiotics and other drugs, including growth hormones.[6]

What is the result of American food-raising practices? You know as well as I do that the most obvious result is an entire population that is over-fed because the United States is the richest country on the face of the earth, and yet which suffers from nutritional deficits and proliferating ailments.

One family at a time, we need to take back the territory we have lost. We need to decide to "eat organic" wherever possible. Essentially, what this means is that we should be choosing to eat in a way that is congruent with the way God designed our bodies. If you do not have a garden of your own, find a local organic farmer who can provide you with local produce. The fresher it is, the better. My family tries to obtain as much as we can from no more than ten miles away from our home.

If you cannot locate a source of organic produce, or if you live in a climate that limits the growth of fruits and vegetables, follow this simple advice: "The best way to shop for food is on the outside perimeter of the grocery store. That is where you will find all of your whole foods: meats, dairy, bread, fruits, and vegetables. When you have done that, *go home!* Everything on the other aisles is sliced, diced, chunked, cooked, and ground foods with chemicals added."[7] Increasingly, supermarkets are establishing special sections (often next to the existing produce department) for organic produce, juices, and other products. These products may cost a little more, but your health is worth it.

FOOD RECOMMENDATIONS

With so many cluttered food pathways available to you, the only way you can navigate your way through the traffic jam is to have some help from someone you trust. Based on natural wellness principles, I would like to make some specific food recommendations to you. (You will find more in Appendix A.)

First let me say that the best approach is always a *positive* one. Instead of focusing on what you cannot eat or should not do, focus on your new goals and your new array of choices. (In DREAM Health, there is no "can't" or "have to," only "choice.")

Having said that, let me also add that your new overall goal is *whole health,* not recovery from illness or improved sex drive or weight loss (fewer chins, less of a spare tire), or happiness in general. All of those benefits will become natural consequences of changing your eating habits and related aspects of your lifestyle.

Always work toward steady, constant improvement and greater balance. Don't make yourself promises you can't keep. Saying you will never eat junk food again is unrealistic for most people. Besides, it's a negative goal, not a positive one. Tell yourself instead that you are going to start keeping fresh, easy-to-grab snacks where you can reach for them.

Recommended vegetables

Eat organically grown vegetables if possible. If not, soak produce in a sink full of water with some organic vegetable wash, distilled vinegar, or 60 drops per gallon of sodium chlorite or hydrogen peroxide. Rinse everything well before eating.

As much as possible, eat your vegetables fresh and raw. If your digestive system reacts with too much bloating, try lightly steaming your vegetables until you get used to the increased vegetable consumption.

Eat as many dark-colored vegetables as possible, and eat as many different colors as possible. Go heavy on the greens and sprouts (eat them as much as you want!), and limit starchy vegetables such as potatoes.

You should purchase a good food scale to keep in your kitchen. Especially where vegetables are concerned, you will be surprised at the sizable portions that you will be serving yourself!

RECOMMENDED VEGETABLES (100-CALORIE SERVING SIZE)

- 25-oz. servings—cucumbers, zucchini, summer squash
- 21-oz. servings—celery, radishes
- 17-oz. servings—Swiss chard, tomatoes, turnips
- 15-oz. servings—asparagus, cabbage, cauliflower, spinach
- 13-oz. servings—broccoli, cauliflower, beet greens, collard greens, sweet peppers, Hubbard squash, kale
- 10-oz. servings—butternut squash, onions, snow peas
- 7-oz. servings—acorn squash, brussels sprouts
- 3-oz. servings—garlic, peas
- 1-oz. servings—avocadoes

ACCEPTABLE VEGETABLES (100-CALORIE SERVING SIZE)

- 21-oz. servings—turnips
- 17-oz. servings—eggplant
- 13-oz. servings—green beans, pumpkin
- 7-oz. servings—beets, leeks, carrots
- 3-oz. servings—yams, parsnips

Recommended fruits

What kinds of fruits grow in the vicinity of your home? When you are looking for fruit, start with your locally grown, organic, or non-sprayed varieties. The advantages of this kind of fruit is that it is more likely to be vine- or tree-ripened, which means it contains more phytochemicals and other health-enhancing qualities, and it is less likely to have been sprayed with the agents that are used to prevent overripening.

But even organically grown fruits are not created equal. Some provide much greater nutritional benefits than others. For instance, I don't recommend melons because they are so high on the glycemic (sugar) index. (This is less true of watermelon.) But I strongly recommend all fruits that are dark in color such as organic blueberries, raspberries, strawberries, blackberries, and cranberries, because they contain higher amounts of antioxidants, especially if they have been grown in good-quality soil.

Once you locate a good fruit source, you can purchase in season and fill your freezer full for the winter months. You will derive greater benefits from your supply of local, vine-ripened fruits than you will from fruits that have been harvested half a continent away and then shipped to your local store. Start your day with a serving of fruit; it's an excellent way to break your overnight fast.

RECOMMENDED FRUITS (100-CALORIE SERVING SIZE):

- 12-oz. servings—lemon juice, lime juice
- 7-oz. servings—blueberries, raspberries, Anjou pears
- 5-oz. servings—blackberries, kiwis, plums

ACCEPTABLE FRUITS (100-CALORIE SERVING SIZE):):

- 12-oz. servings—strawberries (organic only)
- 7-oz. servings—nectarines, peaches, cranberries, green apples
- 5-oz. servings—red apples, grapes, raw figs, bananas
- 1-oz. servings—organic raisins

Nuts and seeds

Nuts and seeds are great sources of both protein and healthy fatty acids. My favorites are almonds, walnuts, Brazil nuts, sunflower seeds, pumpkinseeds, and ground flaxseeds. The oils in nuts and seeds will oxidize when exposed to light, so try to buy them in their shells whenever possible or store them in lightproof containers.

Peanuts are misnamed, because they are not nuts at all, but rather legumes. I don't recommend eating peanuts, as organic peanuts are tainted with the aflatoxin fungus.

As a source of calories, nuts and seeds are denser than fruits and vegetables. The size of a 100-calorie serving of nuts is 2 tablespoons, and the size of a 100-calorie serving of oily nut-butter is only 2 teaspoons.

Recommended meats, fish, and meat substitutes

Remember—the best meats are lean, grass-fed, free-range, and hormone- and antibiotic-free. Unlike grain-fed meats, grass-fed meats will have retained omega-3 fatty acids. Wild game is an excellent source of pure food, although you need to be careful with wild fish, since so many of our oceans and lakes are contaminated with mercury and other pollutants. In Appendix A you will find a listing of mail-order sources for free-range meats and wild game meat.

Organ meats are good for you, *if* they come from hormone- and antibiotic-free animals. I do not recommend organ meats that come from industrially farmed animals.

Lean, fat-trimmed portions of white fish, beef, lamb, game, turkey, and skinless chicken provide about 150–200 calories per 4-ounce serving. Vegetable protein can be used as a substitute for meat.

RECOMMENDED ANIMAL PROTEINS

Caloric values may vary; see www.calorielab.com for more information.

- Wild game—buffalo, deer, elk, caribou, rabbit, etc.
- Red meats—beef, lamb (lean, grass-fed only)
- Fish—wild salmon
- Fowl—chicken and turkey (lean only), wildfowl (pheasant, guinea hen, squab, ostrich, etc.)
- Eggs (free-range only)

ACCEPTABLE ANIMAL PROTEINS

Caloric values may vary; see www.calorielab.com for more information.

- Fish—cod, snapper, rockfish, haddock, halibut, tuna, swordfish (avoid all farmed fish and shellfish)

Grains

In my opinion, grains should be eaten in extreme moderation. Those who feel they just cannot live without grains should choose whole (steel-cut) oats, quinoa, kamut, spelt, amaranth, or organic brown rice in small servings (about ½ cup cooked).

Bread should be limited. (Breads are not whole foods; you don't see bread growing out of the ground, do you?) Those who feel they must eat bread should choose a yeast-free, wheat-free, salt-free version of a whole-grain rye or spelt bread, baked at home, if possible.

And as you are making a food plan, consider carefully what you will put *on* your bread. Is it worth the effort of obtaining good bread if you are going to slather it with mayonnaise and make a bologna sandwich out of it?

Water

As I have already mentioned, water is a foundational item in any healthy diet. Not all of it needs to be consumed as plain water. Enjoy some of your water as it comes in vegetable juices, milks, and fresh produce (although I recommend that you avoid dairy products altogether and use almond milk or rice milk). The best vegetable juices are composed of lots of greens and grasses and sprouts. You might like the taste better if you add a bit of carrot or beet for sweetness. Some ginger and a small amount of garlic can be nice, although don't overdo it—you should make your juices to be enjoyable and not to earn yourself a badge of courage! I don't recommend most fruit juices, with the exception of lemon, lime, and tomato, because of their high glycemic (sugar) content and acid-producing tendencies.

As I already mentioned, your drinking water should be purified; avoid tap water unless you are desperate. Don't assume that bottled water is any better than tap water. Find out how it was processed before you buy it.

At most health food stores, you can get chlorine dioxide or sodium chlorite, which you can add to your water to alkalize it. You can also use hydrogen peroxide for the same purpose, which you can buy at any drugstore or grocery store. Add about five drops per eight-ounce glass of water, and drink your water at room temperature. Easier than these, however, is simply lemon or lime juice, which are my personal favorites.

At least once a day, add a greens mixture to a glass of drinking water. It is a great alkalizer, as well as an excellent source of vitamins and minerals. Green supplements are made from barley grass, wheat grass, oat grass, kamut grass, and lemongrass.

NATURAL RECIPES

Below are some natural recipes that I believe you will find appetizing and enjoyable.[8]

NATURAL DIET VITALITY SMOOTHIE

- 1 cup frozen organic blueberries, raspberries, strawberries, or blackberries
- Lactose-free protein powder (if you don't digest fruit and protein well, try a hemp protein or other vegetable protein or use pre-soaked almonds)
- Organic greens powder
- Organic carrot juice, whole apple juice, almond milk, rice milk, or a combination of any of the above. I like to use carrot juice as my base and add a bit of almond milk for richness
- 1 tsp. of omega-balanced oil (omega 3-6-9)
- 1 Tbsp. ground flaxseed

Put ingredients in a blender or smoothie-maker and whir until all chunks are pureed. I like mine thick enough to eat with a spoon; experiment to see how you prefer yours.

Smoothies are a great place to hide healthy oils and liquid multivitamin and mineral supplements. Your kids will never suspect they're in there if you don't tell them!

Your smoothie should be about 10–12 liquid ounces. It will be calorie-dense, so measure out your portions if you are watching your weight. Limit the total calories to about 400.

NATURAL DIET ORGANIC BIG SALAD

Salad Base
- Organic greens
- Cucumbers

- Peppers, red, green, yellow
- Tomato
- Sprouts, alfalfa, soy, radish, mung bean, if desired
- Seeds

Tear up organic greens and place in serving bowl. Chop or slice cucumbers, peppers, and tomato on top of greens. Top salad with a generous portion of the Vegetable Mix. Top with sprouts and seeds, if you wish. Dress with Natural Diet Vegetable Dressing.

Serving size: *Buy enough giant-size salad bowls so there is one for each member of your family. (Yes, the one you used to put on the table for the whole family is now going to be an individual-size bowl!)*

Vegetable Mix

- Swiss chard
- Kale
- Raw broccoli or cauliflower
- Cabbage
- Carrots
- Celery
- Beets
- Parsley

Combine any of the above ingredients, putting in the whole green leafy vegetable, stem and all. The vegetables should be chopped into pieces about the size of your thumbnail; you can speed up the process by using a food processor.

Put this mixture into a large container (glass is best) that you can seal and keep in the refrigerator. If you wish, sprinkle the mixture with lime or lemon juice or some vitamin C powder to keep it fresh for a longer period. You can add some ginger, onion, or garlic for added flavor.

NATURAL DIET VEGETABLE DRESSING

- 1 tsp. omega-balanced oil or organic flax oil

- 1 tsp. organic extra-virgin cold-pressed olive oil
- Organic lemon or organic (nitrate-free) apple cider vinegar to taste
- Organic seasoning to taste

Put all ingredients in a cruet and shake. Refrigerate. Use with the Natural Diet Organic Big Salad and with other salads.

SUPPLEMENTS

When you buy a box of organic blueberries, or when you pick them yourself straight from the bush, you cannot see the levels of vitamins and other nutrients that may be in those berries. Those nutrient levels will be higher or lower, depending on many factors. How can you tell if you are getting sufficient amounts (or too much) of a particular vitamin or mineral? You *can't* tell, can you?

Besides, regardless of how hard you try to improve your food sources, perfect your meal plans, and handle your food with care, something is sure to be missing. And your personal nutritional needs will vary with your age, gender, activity and stress levels, and your individual health profile.

So what's a conscientious person to do?

The answer is obvious—take supplements. You can ensure your health for years to come by making nutritional supplements a reliable part of your nutritional plan. But ordinary vitamin pills that you can buy at the drugstore aren't good enough. For one thing, pills are more difficult for your body to absorb than are liquid vitamin and mineral supplements. So my recommendation is to take a liquid multivitamin supplement. To make sure that people can obtain a good one, I market my own DREAMHealth Complete supplement. (See the product page at the back of this book.)

Now, no supplement or series of supplements alone can supply all of your nutritional needs. To stay healthy, your body definitely requires whole foods, without which, for instance, you would not consume any fiber. But supplements are an important part of a DREAM Health diet.

Clearly, our ancestors did not take supplements. However, they did eat 100 percent organic food grown in soils that were richer in nutrients than our soil is today. Most of them got lots of fresh air and fresh water. They ate no processed foods, never heard of a food additive or a pesticide, and exercised virtually all day, every day. If we could turn back the clock, and if we could supply ourselves with basic, untainted foods, achieving the healthiest diet possible, taking supplements might become redundant—perhaps even dangerously redundant.

But there is little likelihood of that happening. In reality, it is impossible to eat a totally pure and completely sufficient diet in the industrialized world we find ourselves living in. Today, even organic produce is grown in depleted soils, and most of us lack the time and desire to obtain the large amounts of the right raw vegetables that would be required to match the vitamin, mineral, and fiber needs of an ideal diet. (None of us walk around all day hunting and gathering!)

At the same time, the more fresh vegetables you eat each day, the less you will need to supplement your antioxidant intake. Just as a cut-up apple turns brown and steel exposed to the weather rusts (oxidizes), so the cells of your body can be damaged and destroyed if they are exposed to the chemicals in your outer and inner environment. Antioxidants create a protective barrier around your cells so that they are less vulnerable.

So each one of us needs to take nutritional supplements. In addition to following a "pure and sufficient" eating plan, I strongly recommend that you add the following supplements to your DREAM Health diet:

1. Liquid multivitamin that includes a range of antioxidant vitamins.

2. Balanced fish oil supplement (EPA and DHA) plus balanced omega-3-6-9 fatty acid oil blend (which can be your salad dressing base). Very few people can eat enough fish to ingest an amount of omega-3 fatty acid that will balance out the omega-6 fatty acids that they eat in the form of grains and cereals, and even if they did, their high-fish diet would expose them to the toxicity of mercury, which has been found in every ocean of the world.

3. Multimineral supplement with cell salts ("macrominerals" calcium, magnesium, manganese, zinc, and iron) plus trace minerals such as phosphorous, potassium, selenium, copper, chromium, and iodine. It's good to add extra calcium, magnesium, and potassium.

4. One milligram daily of twelve cell salts (mineral or tissue salts)—calcium fluoride, calcium phosphate, calcium sulfate, ferric phosphate, magnesium sulfate, potassium chloride, potassium phosphate, potassium sulfate, sodium chloride, sodium phosphate, sodium sulfate, and silica. Liquid and colloidal form is best.

5. Balanced B vitamins. Liquid and colloidal form is best.

6. Concentrated greens powder (wheat grass, barley grass, oat grass, kamut grass, lemongrass, plus a variety of vegetable greens). Mix into drinking water or vegetable juice.

7. pH drops for drinking water (chlorine dioxide or sodium chlorite or hydrogen peroxide). If in the typical 2 percent

solution, use five drops per 8-ounce glass of water. You can substitute plain lemon or lime juice.

8. Probiotics

9. Glyconutrients (aloe, mannose, noni juice, etc.)

10. Chromium (for the first year of your new eating plan)

Why do I recommend these particular supplements? Let's take a look at the assortment of vitamins and minerals that your body needs for optimal health.

Vitamins

Vitamins are organic substances essential for the normal growth and vitality of your body. Vitamins help regulate your metabolism, help convert fat and carbohydrates into energy, and assist in forming bone tissue. They also support the biochemical processes that release energy from digested food. Vitamins can be obtained naturally from the foods you eat and from sunshine. In general, your body cannot manufacture its own vitamins, so they must be supplied in your diet or by means of dietary supplements.

Vitamins are either fat-soluble or water-soluble. Fat-soluble vitamins are stored in your fat tissue and in the liver until they are needed. Fat-soluble vitamins include vitamins A, D, E, and K. Water-soluble vitamins are not stored in your body. They travel quickly through your bloodstream, and whatever your body does not use is excreted through your urine. As a result, they must be replaced regularly by means of food or supplements. Water-soluble vitamins include vitamin C and the B vitamins.

Vitamin A enhances night vision; it also regulates the cells of your skin and the lining of your lungs and intestines. The best food sources of vitamin A are eggs, milk, butter, liver, fish, apricots, nectarines, cantaloupe, carrots, spinach, and pumpkin. Vitamin A deficiency is symptomized by night blindness (difficulty seeing at night) and dry or inflamed eyes.

Vitamin D is responsible for forming and maintaining strong bones and teeth. Adequate exposure to sunlight (a few minutes a day in most climates) will help ensure that your body can manufacture enough of the D vitamin. Additional amounts can be supplied through vitamin D fortified milk, cereals, and through tuna and eggs. A vitamin D deficiency is revealed by loss of bone strength (brittle bones).

Vitamin E protects the tissues of your body from damage by free radicals, and it helps your body with vitamin A storage. It also helps the vitamin K blood-clotting function. The best sources of vitamin E are fish oils and vegetable oils such as corn, soy, and peanut. Sunflower seeds, dark leafy green vegetables, and nuts also contain vitamin E in smaller amounts. Symptoms of deficiency include poor muscle coordination, shaky movements, decreased sensitivity to vibration, and general lack of reflexes.

Vitamin K plays an important role in blood clotting. Without vitamin K, any cut in your skin would bleed continuously. Good sources of vitamin K include spinach, lettuce, broccoli, brussels sprouts, cabbage, and cow's milk.

B vitamins are crucial for your nervous system function, and they help your body break down complex carbohydrates into simple sugars so they can be used for energy. B vitamins are also important in metabolic activity and in making red blood cells that carry oxygen throughout your body. Water-soluble B vitamins must be replenished daily.

The best sources of B vitamins are fish, meat, dried beans, breads and cereals, and green leafy vegetables. Symptoms of a possible B vitamin deficiency may include fatigue, reduced secretion of digestive acids, confusion, and forgetfulness.

Vitamin C reaches every cell of your body, and it helps your immune system fight off viral and bacterial invasions, supports the cardiovascular system by protecting tissues from free-radical damage, and assists the health of your nervous system. It is vital to the production of collagen, the fibers of the connective tissue that gives your body form and supports your organs, and it helps wounds to heal. It also helps your body to absorb iron, and it breaks down histamines, the inflammatory component of many allergic reactions.

Vitamin C is abundant in fresh citrus fruits such as oranges, limes, and grapefruit, and in vegetables including tomatoes, green peppers, potatoes, and many others.

Minerals

A mineral is an inorganic element, such as calcium, iron, potassium, sodium, or zinc, that is essential to the nutrition of humans, animals, and plants. Your body uses minerals to perform many different functions, from building strong bones to transmitting nerve impulses to making hormones and maintaining a normal heartbeat.

There are two types of minerals: macrominerals and trace minerals. Macrominerals include calcium, phosphorus, magnesium, sodium, potassium, chloride, and sulfur. They are called macrominerals because your body needs larger amounts of them than it does trace minerals. Trace minerals, as their name implies, are those minerals of which your healthy body requires only a little bit. Trace minerals include iron, manganese, copper, iodine, zinc, cobalt, fluoride, and selenium. Let's explore each of these minerals to find out how important they are to your health.

Calcium helps to build strong bones and healthy teeth. In fact, 99 percent of the calcium in your body is stored in your bones and teeth. Calcium is found primarily in dairy products (milk, yogurt, cheese) and in fortified juices. It is also found in dark green vegetables, nuts, grains, beans, and canned salmon and sardines (if you eat the bones). Calcium deficiency may be signaled by frequent hives, chronic fatigue, canker and cold sores, muscle cramps ("charley horses"), and itchy skin.

Phosphorus works alongside calcium; it is also stored in your bones and teeth. It is important to the maintenance of healthy connective tissues and organs. Since phosphorus is added to processed and refined foods in large quantities, deficiencies of this mineral are rare.

Magnesium supports your bone health, helps in the production of cholesterol, helps to activate many vitamins, and aids in relaxing your muscles. Much of the magnesium in your body (60–65 percent) is stored in your bones. Foods high in magnesium include tofu, beans, fish, green leafy vegetables, nuts, milk, and enriched bread.

Sodium and chloride are required by your body for the regulation of your fluid balance, to help muscles contract, and to conduct nerve impulses. Processed foods generally contain a large amount of sodium. Other sources of sodium include baking soda, table salt, seasonings, and condiments.

Potassium works with sodium and chloride to nourish cells in your body and help keep your blood pressure constant. It also aids nerve impulses and muscle contractions. The best sources for potassium include bananas, avocados, beans, milk products, meat products, and whole grains.

Sulfur helps to maintain elasticity, movement, healing, and repair within your body tissues. It also helps to eliminate muscle, leg, and back cramps. The best food sources of sulfur include red hot peppers, cabbage, brussels sprouts, garlic, onions, and radishes. Symptoms of sulfur deficiency include slow wound healing, brittle nails and hair, gastrointestinal challenges, immune dysfunction, acne, rashes, depression, and memory loss.

Iron is needed for the formation of hemoglobin, the part of the red blood cells that carries oxygen from the lungs to the rest of your body. Foods that are high in iron include liver, red meat, clams, egg yolks, tofu, salmon, molasses, spinach, prunes, raisins, walnuts, cashews, and almonds. Symptoms of iron deficiency include fatigue, irritability, and shortness of breath.

Manganese works as an antioxidant to keep your cellular membranes healthy. It helps to neutralize toxins in your body, and it also helps vitamin C to do its job. The richest sources of manganese are found in whole grains, legumes, nuts, tea, fruits, and vegetables. Manganese deficiency can result in joint pain, high blood sugar, bone or disk problems, and poor memory.

Copper is necessary for proper iron metabolism and for the maintenance of your blood vessels. Copper is also a vital mineral for keeping your skin, blood vessels, and connective tissue supple and elastic. You obtain copper in your diet from seafood, nuts, legumes, and green leafy vegetables.

Iodine helps to metabolize excess fat. It is very important for both mental and physical health, and it is required to keep your thyroid gland functioning normally. A deficiency of this mineral is rare because iodine is added to salt ("iodized salt"). Iodine can also be obtained from bread and seafood.

Zinc is a highly important mineral that is found in every cell of your body. It is involved in many immune mechanisms, and it aids in wound healing. More than three hundred enzymes in the human body require zinc in order to function properly.

You can obtain zinc by consuming beef, poultry, fish, grains, and vegetables. A zinc deficiency is signaled by poor appetite, rough skin, tiredness, and acne.

Selenium is considered an antioxidant, and it plays an important role in your body's enzyme function and immune system. Fish and shellfish, red meat, chicken, liver, grains, eggs, garlic, brewer's yeast, and wheat germ are all good sources for this vital mineral.

NUTRITIONAL HERBS

We take herbs for granted. We use them on a regular basis to flavor our foods, but we don't recognize the fact that they are an important part of a balanced diet. Herbs come from whole plants or their roots, leaves, seeds, and stems. Many herbs are full of vitamins, and they can become natural remedies. Some therapeutic benefits can be traced to specific substances in a plant, but many herbs derive their therapeutic value from dozens of active constituents that work together, which leads many herbalists to recommend the whole plant for its healing properties.

As you know, herbs were the first medicines, and plants are also the original source of many modern-day drugs. Take aspirin, for instance. A related compound is derived from the bark of the white willow tree. The raw material for digitalis is extracted from the foxglove plant. By and large, herbs are safer than prescription or over-the-counter drugs, although toxic reactions are certainly possible.

Herbs occupy a significant role in a balanced, natural diet. Following is an alphabetical list of the most commonly used nutritional herbs.

Alfalfa, an ancient member of the pea family, is grown all over the world as hay feed for livestock, and it is also used in green-food concentrates for humans. Its name, alfalfa, came into English via Spanish and Portuguese from Arabic, Persian, and Kashmiri words that mean "best horse fodder" and "horse power."[9] Most alfalfa derivatives are rich in chlorophyll, vitamins B_6, C, and E, beta-carotene, and calcium, and it is traditionally used as a diuretic, an arthritis remedy, and an aid to weight gain. It may lower blood cholesterol levels and help prevent heart disease and possibly strokes.

Burdock root can be eaten as food or prepared as a tea, in which form it can help to reduce cravings and hunger, thus assisting in weight loss. It is used traditionally to cleanse the blood and to heal the kidneys and liver.

Chamomile, taken as a tea, has long been used to treat anxiety, insomnia, and digestive problems. Studies indicate that the herb is effective at reducing fever, healing wounds and burns (when applied topically), stimulating the immune system, and inducing sleep. Chamomile is nontoxic and gentle enough for use with children.

Cinnamon, in preliminary studies at the Human Nutrition Research Center on Aging at Tufts University in Boston, has been found to increase the ability of insulin to metabolize blood sugar, even when ingested in very small daily doses.[10] Therefore, it can be used to protect against the effects of diabetes, reduce hunger, and help control sugar cravings.

Comfrey has traditionally been taken internally as a digestive aid. It has also been discovered to promote cell regeneration and to help relieve inflammation resulting from bruises, sprains, insect bites, and skin conditions.

Cumin, a spice widely used throughout the Middle East, lowers blood cholesterol and inhibits platelet aggregation, both of which protect against heart disease. Scientists in Israel have found that people who eat regular amounts of cumin evidence lower numbers of urinary tract cancers.

Dandelion is high in nutrients, including beta-carotene, vitamin C, and potassium. Traditionally, dandelion leaves (in tea) have been used as a diuretic, and both the leaf and root have been used to treat liver, gallbladder, and kidney ailments and to help improve digestion and rheumatism. They are also considered a mild laxative. It is safe and nontoxic in its preparations.

Garlic, widely used in cooking (although heat inactivates its enzymes and significantly reduces its beneficial effects), is a rich source of protein, vitamins A, B complex, and C, and various trace minerals. Researchers have discovered more than two hundred compounds in garlic, and it is proving to be useful in the treatment or prevention of heart disease. In addition, garlic is a natural antibiotic, antifungal, and antiviral that can be used internally or externally.

Ginger is beneficial for its calming effect on the digestive system and is therefore used as a natural remedy for nausea, upset stomach, and motion sickness. It helps expel gas from the intestines and relaxes and soothes the intestinal tract. It may also lower blood cholesterol levels and lessen the chance of heart attacks and strokes.

Green tea, taken either in capsule form or as a beverage, provides numerous health benefits. It contains chemical compounds called polyphenols, which are not present in the more common black teas and which act as powerful antioxidants. People who drink five cups of green tea a day may have a resulting lower risk of suffering from cancer, heart attacks, and strokes, as well as lower incidence of gum disease and cavities. The polyphenols in green tea also attack the bacteria that cause bad breath.

Kelp is among the richest sources of the element iodine, which is required by the thyroid hormones to regulate the growth and development of a growing human body. Kelp is generally used as a condiment and nutritional supplement.

Licorice is naturally sweet and is used in candies, herbal combination products, and other foods. It is used to relieve respiratory problems, treat ulcers, alleviate arthritis, and control liver conditions.

Mint, such as spearmint and peppermint, is high in calcium, vitamins A and C, riboflavin, and trace minerals. It aids digestion and helps to prevent insomnia, upset stomachs, nasal stuffiness, and nervous tension. Many people like to drink mint tea after meals.

Parsley is full of vitamins A, B, and C, plus iron, iodine, and magnesium. As a result, it stimulates the immune system and strengthens your body's iron count.

Rose hips are often the source of vitamin C in natural supplements. In the form of tea or supplements, their high vitamin C content and bioflavonoids help to keep the response of your immune system healthy.

Rosemary is a popular cooking herb that has a positive effect on your nervous and circulatory systems. It has been used to treat chronic circulatory weaknesses such as low blood pressure. It stimulates the appetite, aids digestion, and works as an antioxidant. Rosemary should be avoided in pregnancy.

HOW OFTEN SHOULD YOU EAT?

It's all very well to learn so much about the detailed pros and cons of various foods and supplements. The big question remains: How often should you eat? Three times a day?

Instead of eating three "squares" a day, I suggest eating five or six small meals throughout the day. Your meals should start first thing in the morning, with breakfast. People who are overweight typically skip breakfast, eat a lunch of processed foods, eat a dinner of processed foods, and then snack on processed foods after dinner until bedtime. Not only are they missing out on being well-fueled and sharp all morning, they are also missing a wonderful way to start up their body's metabolism and to keep it working throughout the day. A high-functioning metabolism translates into burned calories. Oatmeal is a natural for breakfast, and it goes well with fruit. I eat mine with nuts and raisins, and locally grown honey (which is an old homeopathic remedy for allergies) on the side.

To keep your metabolism functioning in high gear all day long, follow your breakfast with a midmorning snack of fruit and nuts, a lunch of vegetables and fruit or a salad with sliced chicken breast or tuna, a midafternoon snack of sliced chicken breast and/or nuts and fruit, and a dinner of cooked vegetables and raw salad vegetables served with fish, chicken, or lean beef.

At our house, my wife makes the fresh veggies easy to grab for a snack. Once a week she cuts up broccoli, red sweet peppers, celery, radishes, and jicama root, and she keeps them fresh in a big Tupperware container. So all week long, when our children or one of us feels like snacking, we can just go to the fridge and "grab some purity." It's all in the preparation. If you have such foods easily available, you will choose them. We all find it easiest to eat what's in front of us.

My philosophy is to eat as often as six times daily, but to confine my choices to healthy ones. Then I do not eat after 8:00 p.m., when it is important to give my body time to catch up, assimilate what I have eaten during the day, and rest. Cardiologist William Gavin recommends that people should not eat anything "white" at night. He writes, "White translates to starchy carbohydrates, no matter their color—pasta, rice, potatoes, bread, corn, beans."[11] The reason for "no white at night" is that your body uses starchy foods for either energy or stores them as fat, and since we have limited physical activity in the evening, the energy from the starchy foods will most likely be stored as fat, which is an undesirable outcome.

TRANSITIONING TO A NEW WAY OF EATING

No one can take the information in this chapter and instantly reform his "eating life." Too many changes too fast will spell discouragement and failure. What's the best way to change to a new way of eating? Answer: take it easy and slow. As you choose what to put in your body, filter your choices through the lens of toxicity and deficiency. For starters, choose one or two of these ideas, and make them a part of your daily life:

- Increase the amount of water you drink (with greens or lemon or lime juice and/or pH drops).

- Eat some raw vegetables or fruit with every meal.

- Try to eat smaller meals, five to six times a day; make lunch or breakfast your biggest meal.

- Take recommended supplements.

- Drink some vegetable juice every day.

- Eat grass-fed meats.

- Make your own salad dressings out of healthful oils and other ingredients.

- For one week, measure all of your food portions and count the calories for each food group.

As you become accustomed to several of these changes, you may decide to implement a three-stage approach to further changes.

Changing from processed foods to whole foods

1. First, reduce your intake of highly processed foods.

2. Then begin to choose at least 70 percent of your foods from whole, natural sources.

3. Finally, eliminate your intake of highly processed foods.

Changing your breakfasts

1. At first, simply take vitamin and fish oil supplements, and eat your regular breakfast. You could add ½ cup of

organic vegetable juice and one serving of fresh or frozen fruit. (If you used to skip breakfast, simply starting to eat in the morning would be a big change.)

2. After a while, try eating a breakfast of oatmeal and eggs plus ½ cup of organic vegetable juice and one serving of fresh or frozen fruit. Also, take your vitamin and fish oil supplements.

3. Finally, transition to starting your day with ½ cup of carrot juice with organic greens powder, followed with a Natural Diet Vitality Smoothie (page 63) for breakfast. Make sure that it includes vegetable juice, and don't forget to take your vitamin and fish oil supplements.

Changing your lunches

1. Eat your choice of foods, but incorporate some raw vegetables and lean protein.

2. Make yourself a Natural Diet Organic Big Salad and Dressing (page 63) or steamed vegetables with protein.

3. Eat unlimited portions of low-glycemic vegetables (with seeds OK), plus 150 calories of Natural Diet Vegetable Dressing. Eat 300 calories of approved animal protein, or an unsweetened lactose-free protein drink or hemp protein or other vegetable protein.

Changing your dinners

1. Eat the dinner of your choice, incorporating some raw or steamed vegetables as well as protein. Use Natural Diet Vegetable Dressing (page 64) on your dinner salad.

2. Make a Natural Diet Organic Big Salad (page 63) or other big salad as your main dish. Incorporate some protein and dress it with Natural Diet Vegetable Dressing.

3. Eat unlimited portions of low-glycemic vegetables (with seeds OK), plus 150 calories of Natural Diet Vegetable Dressing. Eat 300 calories of approved animal protein or an unsweetened lactose-free protein drink or hemp protein or other vegetable protein.

A WORD ABOUT EATING OUT

I would be remiss if I didn't address one particular aspect of the twenty-first-century American lifestyle: eating out. Even if you eat in restaurants only occasionally, you need to think about how you can maintain your healthy eating patterns when your choices are limited to what is on the menu.

Naturally, it makes sense to see if you can locate restaurants that offer the healthiest choices. Many fine establishments cater to people who are interested in eating more wholesome foods. Choose eating places that offer a salad bar, broiled and vegetarian foods, and low-fat foods. But in almost every restaurant you can find some healthy options, especially if you ask questions, monitor your portion sizes, and ask for substitutions.

As you read the menu, look for the terms "baked," "broiled," "grilled," "poached," "roasted," or "steamed." Depending on the type of oil used, "sautéed" or "stir-fried" might also be all right. Avoid menu items that include the terms "fried," "alfredo," "au gratin," "breaded," "buttered," "creamed," "hollandaise," "fricasséed," and "deep-fat fried."

Even if you are celebrating a special occasion, you can make the most of your time with your companion or your family by eating healthfully and well.

Tips for eating out

- Avoid fried or breaded appetizers or main dishes.

- Order vegetables, fruits, and fish.

- With a baked potato, ask for salsa (low in fat and full of good ingredients) instead of sour cream, butter, cheese, or bacon.

- Avoid cream-based soups or chowder. Choose broth-based or tomato-based soups instead.

- Order salad dressings on the side, and watch out for salads that have lots of extras such as cheeses, eggs, and meat.

- For your beverage, order water with lemon or decaffeinated tea.

- Choose whole-grain breads and rolls.

- Order your sandwiches with mustard instead of mayonnaise. Mustard is a flavorful, low-fat alternative.

- Choose low-fat side dishes such as steamed vegetables, a plain baked potato, or a green salad (with dressing on the side) instead of french fries or coleslaw.

- Cut your portion in half and share it with your companion, or take it home for another meal.

- For dessert, order fresh fruit, gelatin, angel food cake, or sherbet. If you want to enjoy the occasional piece of chocolate mousse, share your portion with someone.

Brown-bag it! When you are trying to eat nutritious foods, workday lunches can be your downfall. If you are able to eat at all, often it seems that your lunch must be take-out food gobbled at your desk or in your car.

Do you have a refrigerator at your workplace? If so, stock it on Monday with items you can eat throughout the week, such as yogurt, fruits, vegetables, low-fat cheeses, and juices. Keep an area in a desk drawer stocked with healthy foods such as nuts, whole-grain bread or crackers, a jar of peanut butter, popcorn (minus heavy salt and butter), rice cakes, and good quality canned soups.

Most practical of all, pack yourself a brown-bag lunch every day. (The time you would have used to drive to buy your lunch can be better spent taking a refreshing walk!) The hand-packed contents of your lunch will give you energy for the rest of your workday.

What can you put into your brown bag? A good rule of thumb is to include at least one fruit and one vegetable in your lunch every day. Here are some other healthful choices for your brown-bag lunches:

- Make a sandwich on whole-grain bread, a pita pocket, a bagel, or an English muffin.

- Make sandwich fillings from lean, organic turkey, chicken, ham, or tuna, along with avocado slices, tomato, and lettuce.

- Pack a container of raw vegetables and fruit.

- Include a bottle or can of 100 percent fruit or vegetable juice.

- Bring cut-up fruits or vegetables with a yogurt dip.

- Make some vegetarian burritos.

- Make a low-fat pasta salad.

- Bring a banana, and eat it with some almond butter.

- Prepare a garden salad with a variety of vegetables.

LOOKING BACK

Optimal health requires optimal nutrition. As you apply what you are learning about how, when, and what to eat and drink, you will feel better and stay healthier.

Although you may be starting from what I call the "American Death Diet," you can change to a whole-foods diet that is as balanced and achievable as it is varied and enjoyable. Start with making just one change to your diet, such as adding valuable supplements, including more fruits and vegetables, buying more organic foods, or drinking more water. As you begin to feel more alert and healthy, you will find it easier to make further changes.

It is imperative that you start looking at your food as nutrition that you choose because it is congruent with the design of your body, not just empty-calorie fuel. You do this by asking yourself two questions: Is the food I am putting into my body toxic, or is it pure? Am I deficient in something, or am I sufficient in it? If you learn to view your nutrition decisions through this lens, your diet and other lifestyle patterns will change.

☑ TO-DO LIST

☑ Go through your kitchen and take stock of how many simple carbohydrates (white flour, white rice, sugar-containing products) you have on hand. Choose which ones you are going to reduce or eliminate from your diet.

☑ Eat more whole, unrefined foods.

☑ Eat smaller, more frequent meals.

☑ Invest in good vitamin, mineral, and omega-3 supplements.

☑ Consume more nutritional herbs.

☑ Decide to stop snacking after 8:00 p.m.

Rest: Vital to Your Health

⌒⌒

Sleep is the golden chain that ties health and our bodies together.

—THOMAS DEKKER

⌒⌒

The *R* of DREAM Health stands for *rest*. You and I will never achieve and sustain our health unless we get adequate daily rest, much of it in the form of restful sleep. When we rest, our bodies and minds shut down, allowing them to regenerate and heal.

Instinctively we know how important rest is. Remember the classic Benjamin Franklin proverb? "Early to bed and early to rise makes a man healthy, wealthy, and wise." In this chapter I will tell you how essential rest is to your overall health and how to get the best rest possible, so that your whole life can flow better than ever.

In his book *Healing by Design: Unlocking Your Body's Potential to Heal Itself,* Dr. Scott Hannen writes:

> The body was designed to work hard, but it was also designed to rest and to heal. If the body consistently receives the proper

amount of rest, it will have adequate time to heal. Then the body is prepared for the work you face the next day. The problem is that in our "microwave society," everything moves at such a fast pace that it appears to be nonstop, and the body never gets a chance for rest or recovery from the continual stimuli that place stress on it.[1]

LONG DAYS, SHORT NIGHTS

So many of us—and this may include you—work long days at stressful jobs and do not know what a difference it would make to get enough sleep. We may hardly ever take naps, and we may not even take real breaks during the day to "recharge our batteries." We may take the occasional vacation, but too often discover that our vacations are filled with as much activity as we have in our daily working lives. This puts our bodies under chronic stress. Physiologically, we were not designed to be under chronic stress, but rather only short-term stress.

> *A good laugh and a long sleep are the best cures in the doctor's book.*
>
> —IRISH PROVERB

Most of us work hard to support and take care of our families and other people, which means that we take care of ourselves last. I'm going to ask you to reverse your approach. Think about the last time you flew in an airplane. As a safety precaution, the flight attendant advised you that if an emergency situation should arise and the oxygen masks should drop down in front of you, you should secure your own mask before attending to others. The reason for this advice is, of course, to prevent you from losing consciousness, in which case you would be unable to assist anyone else, not to mention unable to take care of yourself further.

In this same way, I believe that by taking care of yourself first, you will be much better able to support everyone else in your life.

You will be a better spouse, a better parent, a better employee or employer—everything in your life will work better. You will be able to accomplish more work with more energy, and you will feel less fatigue at the end of the day.

A good rest is half the work.

—YUGOSLAVIAN PROVERB

SWEET SLEEP

Sleep allows your body to heal and your cells to grow and repair. It also allows your mind to rest and helps your body to fight infection. When you are fully rested, you are able to think more clearly and perform better physically. Sleep allows your hormone levels to balance, specifically the hormone serotonin, which is a major player in mood and depression.

The amount of sleep you get is likely to play a significant role in your ability to stick with a moderate, nutritious diet. When you feel tired, you are more likely to eat just to stay awake or to obtain energy or just satisfy your fatigued body with whatever is in front of you, whether it is toxic or not. According to fitness expert Jorge Cruise, "Lack of sleep...affects your levels of leptin, the hormone that makes you feel full. When levels are low, you crave sweets such as candy, desserts, and even starches. Lack of sleep can also slow your metabolism, which prevents your body from using glucose effectively."[2]

In a widely distributed news service article, Dr. Michael Thorpy, director of the Sleep-Wake Disorders Center at Montefiore Medical Center in New York City, stated:

> Studies show that if people get less sleep than they should, that this affects various components of metabolism. A number of different hormones affect metabolism and can affect appetite and

therefore weight. Blood glucose tends to be higher, insulin levels lower and cortisol levels higher after sleep deprivation. There's additional evidence that the hormone leptin (secreted by fat cells) is influenced by sleep loss, and there are some studies that are...showing that people after sleep loss have an increase in appetite, so they eat more.[3]

Most of us would be quick to say that we want to eat right and want to be more energetic and healthy. (No one in their right mind would wish to be poorly nourished, fatigued, and sick!) Yet how do we expect to accomplish this without making every effort to get a full night's sleep?

Somehow we consider sleep to be an interruption to more valuable activities, even a waste of time. We try all kinds of ways to pump up our energy level with caffeine, drugs, and sugar, all the while stubbornly refusing to simply lie down and rest. We lose our ability to listen to the message our tired bodies are trying to give us.

Unfortunately, the effects of getting too little rest often don't show up for years. Our bodies, which must struggle to repair themselves with too little rest, begin to break down little by little. We make poor choices because we don't feel like exercising or eating what's good for us. We become clumsy and may sustain injuries. We may fall ill. Our rest-deprived bodies rack up additional stresses on a daily basis, which keep us from recovering.

Human beings can live about five minutes without air, three days without water, and a month without food. No one has ever perished solely due to lack of sleep, because the human body, after being severely sleep-deprived, will defy circumstances in order to snatch mini-naps. Drowsy driving, one of the most common results of sleep deprivation, has been reported as the cause of at least 100,000 accidents, 71,000 injuries, and 1,550 fatalities in the United

States each year.[4] Sleep is essential—without it, we cannot survive. With too little of it, our quality of life is severely compromised.

Sleep deprivation

Many of us do not even realize that we are sleep-deprived because we don't know what it feels like to be fully rested. Most healthy adults require about eight hours of solid, restful sleep daily in order to remain healthy and productive. However, very few people get that much sleep.

How much sleep do you get on an average weeknight? I believe that for every hour of sleep that you have come short of the eight hours of recommended sleep, it will take you two extra hours of sleep to replenish what you lost. Replacing your sleep deficiency with sleep sufficiency is harder than getting enough sleep in the first place.

And it's not just a matter of making up for lost down time—if we don't address our sleep deprivation, it increases our stress response, which you read about in chapter three. Chronic stress leads to all kinds of ailments. Suddenly, your lack of sleep has become a culprit in your high blood pressure or your diabetes.

You see, your sleep is like an essential nutrient of your diet. If you don't get enough of it, you will develop disease, just as people who don't get enough vitamin C develop scurvy. But if you replace your deficiency of sleep with sufficiency, the natural healing process of your body can work much better. Your body gets what it needs to move toward continued health, without any outside medical intervention.

The National Sleep Foundation reports that the average American adult sleeps 6.8 hours on weekday nights and 7.4 hours on weekend nights.[5] Another NSF poll also reveals that teenagers, who require more sleep than adults, are not getting enough sleep. "Overall, 45% of adolescents get an insufficient amount of sleep on school nights (less than 8 hours). In addition, about three in ten (31%) get a borderline amount of sleep (8 to less than 9 hours). This leaves only 20% of adolescents getting the optimal amount of sleep (9 hours or more)."[6]

Safety issues

The National Sleep Foundation reports that in the past century, we have reduced our average time asleep by 20 percent, and in the past 25 years, added a month to our average annual work-commute time.[7]

When a person is sleep-deprived, his overall safety is affected, especially on the highway, although, as reported by the National Highway Traffic Safety Administration, determining which accidents were caused by sleep deprivation is not as easy as determining, for instance, which accidents are caused by alcohol consumption.

Unlike the situation with alcohol-related crashes, no blood, breath, or other objective test for sleepiness currently exists that is administered to a driver at the scene of a crash. No definitive criteria are available for establishing how sleepy a driver is or a threshold at which driver sleepiness affects safety. If drivers are unharmed in a crash, hyperarousal following the crash usually eliminates any residual impairment that could assist investigating officers in attributing a crash to sleepiness.

As a result, our understanding of drowsy-driving crashes is based on subjective evidence, such as police crash reports and driver self-reports following the event, and may rely on surrogate measures of sleepiness, such as duration of sleep in a recent time-frame or sleep/work patterns. Some researchers have addressed the problem by analyzing only those crashes known not to be caused by alcohol (because alcohol can cause sleepiness and affect other performance variables), mechanical problems, or other

factors and by looking for evidence of a sleepiness effect in categories of inattention or fatigue.[8]

Estimates of the number of fatigue-caused accidents, nevertheless, are revealing. The National Highway Traffic Safety
Administration estimates that sleepiness results in as many as one
hundred thousand car crashes per year.[9]

Other safety issues are also greatly affected by sleep deprivation.
Dr. Carl Hunt, director of the National Center on Sleep Disorders
Research, declares, "We are all affected by sleep problems. Even if
you personally get sufficient sleep to feel refreshed each day, chances
are you interact with someone who has a sleep problem. It could be
your mother, whose sleep apnea increases her chances of developing
heart disease; your carpool driver, who might be at increased risk
for a car crash because of poor sleep; or your child, who has trouble
in school because she doesn't get enough sleep at night."[10]

A study reported in the January 27, 2003, issue of the *Archives of
Internal Medicine* followed 71,617 professional women over a ten-year
period, looking for a correlation between hours of sleep and risk of
coronary heart disease. The study results showed that women who
slept five hours or less per night faced a 30 percent increased risk of
coronary heart disease than those who slept nine hours per night.
Sleeping an average of six hours per night was associated with an
18 percent greater risk.[11] This supports my point about how our
increased stress response due to lack of sleep increases disease.

Many studies have been conducted to show the effects of sleep
deprivation on job performance. Minor performance errors are relatively insignificant, but sometimes sleep deprivation can have disastrous effects. Dr. Gerald Rosen, sleep specialist from the University
of Minnesota, reports that "disasters such as Chernobyl, Three
Mile Island, Challenger, Bhopal, and Exxon Valdez were officially
attributed to errors in judgment induced by sleepiness or fatigue."[12]

Closer to home, shift workers, who comprise 20 percent of the workforce in the United States, suffer from what sleep researchers call "blue collar jet lag." Dr. Rosen reports that 55 percent of night shift workers describe nodding off or falling asleep at work at least once a week. As many as 30 percent of them report that this occurs more than three times a week. Additionally, 25 percent of shift workers, especially those who work at night, say they tend to fall asleep while they are operating equipment. In Dr. Rosen's words, "Sleep is not negotiable. It is a biological imperative."[13]

How do you know if you are sleep-deprived? Obviously, if you are sleepy and tired most of the time, you should suspect that you're not getting adequate rest through sleep. According to the Web site Helpguide, one or more of the following signs indicate that you should get more sleep:

- Difficulty waking up in the morning
- Inability to concentrate
- Falling asleep during work or class
- Feelings of moodiness, irritability, depression, or anxiety[14]

HOW TO GET GOOD SLEEP

I hope we have established that sleep is an essential part of wholeness.

Do you realize that you have already spent *years* of your life sleeping? How old are you? You have spent one-third of those years lying down. For that reason alone, it is vital to maximize the benefits of your sleeping time.

We all know that the number of hours we spend in our beds doesn't necessarily mean we are getting that number of hours of high-quality sleep. A truly restful night's sleep occurs when you stay sleeping through a number of complete sleep cycles, which run from ninety minutes to one hundred ten minutes, becoming longer as the night progresses. About 20 percent of your night is spent in REM (rapid eye movement) sleep, which is when you are dreaming. Toward morning, if you sleep long enough, almost all of your sleep is restorative REM sleep.[15] The obvious goal is to sleep soundly for long enough to get the full benefits of the sleep process.

Sleep posture

Even if you are trying to sleep the recommended eight hours a night, you won't sleep soundly if you are uncomfortable, and you won't wake up refreshed if you sleep in a contorted position.

The best sleeping posture is to sleep on your back with a good pillow supporting your neck and your spine straight (as if you were standing), or on your side with your knees pulled up, possibly with a small pillow between your legs for comfort. A facedown posture compounds back problems by exaggerating the curvature of your lower back. When you sleep on your stomach, you also must turn your face to one side in an unnatural position, which places undue stress on your neck and spine.

Do you wake up with aches and pains in your body? Do you slouch when you're standing or sitting? Dr. Burle Pettibone, an expert in spinal posture, states that 90 percent of spinal stress occurs from our sleeping posture.[16] You may not realize how many different sleep positions you adopt over the course of a night, but you probably know your favorite position. Perhaps you should take a look at your typical sleep positions, because making improvements in your sleep posture will help you stand, sit, and feel better when you are awake.

Good body support

What you sleep on is as important as how long you sleep and your habitual sleep posture.

For proper support and sleep-enhancing comfort, I recommend a good spring coil mattress or a visco-elastic, high-density foam mattress. The latter was originally created by NASA for use in the space program. The foam senses body weight and temperature and automatically adjusts its support, which relieves the uncomfortable pressures that cause a person to toss and turn during the night. I also recommend 100 percent cotton bedding, because it "breathes" and keeps you more comfortable.

Should you use sleep aids?

When the typical American adult has problems sleeping, too often he or she looks for a solution at the drugstore. Sleep-inducing drugs may knock you out for a night, but they do not address the underlying problems, and they are likely to add a few problems of their own.

Those side effects include chemical addiction, memory loss, mental confusion, and stomach problems, and they can occur if you take either over-the-counter sleep aids, such as Nytol and Sominex, or prescription sleeping pills, such as Halcion, Dalmane, Valium, Restoril, Ambien, and Seconal. Benzodiazepines (Dalmane and Valium are the most widely prescribed) are particularly implicated in mental impairment side effects. Although they are prescribed to aid sleep, they seem to interfere with the crucial REM stage of sleep, which is so crucial to overall alertness and health.[17] In addition, benzodiazepines may do damage to your bones. They have been associated with an increased risk of osteoporosis-related hip fractures.[18]

Along with many other wellness advisors, including psychiatry professor Daniel Kripke of the University of California/San Diego, I also believe we should "wake up" to the fact that sleeping pills are unsafe in any amount.[19] I believe that you should not take sleeping pills, including over-the-counter pills and melatonin.

HOW TO GET BETTER SLEEP

- Catch up on your sleep. Go to sleep earlier and sleep in a little later than normal.
- Take a nap whenever you don't feel rested.
- Increase the number of hours you sleep each week by setting a bedtime for yourself that is at least an hour earlier than you normally go to bed.
- Get some exercise every day. Even a short walk will help you sleep later on.
- Make sure you have fresh air in the room where you sleep.
- Choose 100 percent cotton bedding.
- Consider natural supplements that are known to aid sleep, such as the curry spice turmeric, chamomile, passionflower, kava kava, hops, valerian, St. John's Wort, calcium, and magnesium. (Check with your health-care provider first.)
- Try stress-reducing techniques, including the simple strategy of taking a warm, relaxing bath just before you go to bed.
- Listen to relaxing music either during the day or before bedtime.
- Reduce the distractions in your sleeping area. Especially consider removing a television set or a working area from the bedroom.
- Watch out for caffeine and other stimulants in over-the-counter medications and herbal remedies. This includes ginseng and licorice.

Instead of drugging yourself to sleep, I recommend that you consider the following:

1. If you have trouble getting to sleep, don't go to bed until you are sleepy.

2. Get up at the same time every morning, even after a bad night's sleep. The next night, you'll be sleepy at bedtime.

3. If you wake up in the middle of the night and can't fall back to sleep, get out of bed and return only when you feel sleepy.

4. Keep your bed for sleeping only. Avoid reading (especially thrillers), watching TV, and fretting about your life circumstances. If you want to read thrillers or watch TV, sit in a chair that's not in your bedroom.

5. Avoid alcohol as a sleep aid. It's relaxing at first, but insomnia can result when it clears your system.

6. Avoid drinking or eating anything caffeinated within six hours of your bedtime.

7. Spend time outdoors. People sleep better after they have been exposed to daylight or to bright light therapy.[20]

WHAT ABOUT NAPPING?

In the National Sleep Foundation's 2005 Sleep in America poll, more than one-half of the respondents (55 percent) said they take, on average, at least one nap during the week. One-third (35 percent) of the people polled reported that they take two or more naps a week.[21]

I highly recommend napping. In fact, like the people in many other cultures, I follow a routine of taking a daily fifteen-minute nap. This is in addition to my full, restful night of sleep. My short naptime works wonders!

It took me a solid six months to train myself to do this, but the good results have been well worth my persistent effort. Although some people find it difficult to fall asleep in the middle of the day, I have found that taking a nap can be learned with practice. It's like any other habit. You can train yourself to shut down your brain for fifteen minutes a day.

Even at work, you can lean back in your chair, close your eyes in your car at lunchtime, or lie down on a couch if it is available. Some employers provide their workers with a "quiet" room or a "rest" room on the premises of the workplace. These employers realize that their workforce will be more productive if they can take a break to recharge. With a good rest time built into the workday, people can relate better to their co-workers and to the public, they can be more creative, and they will also be more careful and safety-conscious.

During a nap, your hormone levels rebalance, improving your mood and reducing your stress level. You can relax from the pressures of the morning and get rejuvenated for the demands of the afternoon. In my experience, it is much easier to get through two short half-days of work than it is to get through one long, full day.

Naturally, you shouldn't lie down too close to your bedtime. Nor should you sleep more than an hour and a half, because doing that will throw off your body's circadian rhythm, the internal clock that tells you whether you should be sleeping or not.

If you start taking a little siesta every afternoon, I guarantee that you will reap benefits in your overall health.

VACATION TIME

Many of us work forty, sixty, even eighty hours per week, barely taking lunch breaks, let alone taking a long weekend once in a while. Statistically, large numbers of Americans are working more hours than ever, including the work they do in their own homes, in spite of so-called "time-saving" advances.

Workload, leisure time activities, and proliferating technology combine to create an information overload that is unparalleled in human history. A twenty-first-century American takes in more information from one Sunday *New York Times* than the average person two hundred years ago ingested in a lifetime. Every office and most of our homes have access to the Internet around the clock, and most people carry cell phones that allow them to be on-call virtually all of the time. We are bombarded with information!

What can we do about this? We can't turn back progress, and most of us can't retire early. But we certainly can't keep up this pace indefinitely without a respite. We need to rest. We need vacations.

If your workplace offers vacation days, you would be well-advised to take advantage of them. Even if you are self-employed, you can take days off. Dr. Susan Neal, an Austin-based organization development consultant, writes:

> It's important for each of us to take the time out to care for ourselves. That means paying attention to all of our needs, physical, mental, psychological and spiritual.
>
> The more balanced people can be in all these areas, the more creativity and fresh perspective they have to bring to their work. It's an energy thing. If you are depleted of energy, then you're not good to anyone, most of all yourself. Taking the time off available from their employers can be very positive for the employees and everyone they interact with at home and at work.[22]

No matter what your work situation is like, you need to make it a priority to get away from your daily grind—and from the information overload that threatens to overwhelm you. You need to recharge your physical, mental, and spiritual batteries.

An annual, weeklong vacation will not be enough. You also need to take mini-vacations throughout the year. I try to make sure that I get at least one long weekend off per month, when I spend time with my wife and children. Of course, I also spend time with them on other weekends and weekdays, but this long weekend is extra "us" time. We let go of the busyness of our lives and just enjoy each other. These times furnish the balance that is so important and so hard to achieve without getting away.

On these weekends and on my longer vacations, I like to say that I "lay in the mud like a rhino." A rhino takes great pleasure in wallowing in the mud, often with other rhinos. The mud helps to cool down their bodies (which de-stresses them), protect them from insects (which lets them escape from irritations), and provide sunscreen for them (which protects them).

I know many of you are saying, "There is absolutely no way I can work this many vacations into my schedule." Maybe not right away. But if you make it a goal, you may be surprised at the creative ways you can set up your circumstances in order to make it possible, even in our fast-paced and goal-driven society.

DE-STRESS YOURSELF

Meditation

Most of us never quit thinking throughout the entire day. Our minds churn along constantly, and we can hardly distinguish our thinking processes from our breathing.

But thinking can be turned on and off, and you can "change the channel." It's a bit like a computer program. Our thinking function can be turned on as our situation requires, and then it can be turned down or off so that we can be free and relaxed. Of course we should use our God-given intelligence as responsible stewards of the things God has given us to take care of. But it is equally OK to just "let go and let God."

When I talk about meditation, I am simply talking about quiet and focused thinking that brings my human spirit into a connection with God's Spirit. When I am connected to God, I am not stressed about anything. I am not wearing myself out the way I do when my brain is busy. I am free to consider the important things in life, such as who I am, what my purpose is in life, what I want to become.

I have developed the habit of taking time for quiet meditation every day, because the benefits flow over into the rest of my day (and night). As has been well documented, meditation can help to lower blood pressure, reduce anxiety, lower oxygen consumption, increase blood flow, slow the heart, decrease muscle tension, decrease cholesterol levels, and improve the flow of air to the lungs. Regular meditation even enhances the immune system.

When I take a time of meditation, I go to a quiet environment where I can be undistracted. I wear clothing that is comfortable. I have found it to be helpful, although it's not required, to have a corner of a room or a favorite chair set aside for consistent use. I need a good, comfortable upright position (not lying down, lest I fall asleep) in which I can relax while holding my spine straight.

I have learned to use what is termed "abdominal breathing," which differs from the kind of shallow breathing that most of us do automatically. Try it: take a large breath in, one that is big enough to expand your abdominal area as well as your chest. Make your belly button stick out. After several of these deep breaths, you will notice that your muscles will start to relax. You can continue in this way, inhaling oxygen for health and exhaling all of your stresses, worries, and cares.

My meditation is not passive. While I shut off the flow of self-initiated thinking in my brain, I remain in a state of quiet listening. I am listening for the "still, small voice" of God's Spirit. I am not "emptying" my mind; I am "renewing" it as Paul instructs us to do. (See Romans 12:2.)

Prayer

Prayer and meditation go hand-in-hand. St. John Climacus (525–605 A.D.), who spent his whole life in prayerful contemplation, said, "Prayer is...an expiation of sin, a bridge across temptation a bulwark against affliction. It wipes out conflict, is the work of angels, and is the nourishment of everything spiritual."[23]

You can pray anywhere, anytime. Robert A. Schuller covers the wide range of possibilities:

> Prayer can be practiced in a number of ways. You can pray while driving to work, walking the dog, or resting in bed. It can be done on your knees, on your feet, or flat on your back....Some people pray silently. Others shout. I have been to a Korean church in which everyone prays aloud at the same time for about five minutes until an elder rings a bell signaling that it is time to stop. At the Wailing Wall in Jerusalem, many Jews chant their prayers while rocking back and forth....There is no one way or method of prayer that is necessarily better than another. The important thing is to pray.[24]

The apostle Paul wrote:

> Do not be anxious about anything, but in everything, by prayer and petition, with thanksgiving, present your requests to God. And the peace of God, which transcends all understanding, will guard your hearts and your minds in Christ Jesus....Whatever is true, whatever is noble, whatever is right, whatever is pure, whatever is lovely, whatever is admirable—if anything is excellent or praiseworthy—think about such things.
>
> —PHILIPPIANS 4:6–9

Prayer helps us to recharge our spiritual batteries, gain strength and wisdom, and deepen our spiritual growth. When we pray, we gain access to the Spirit of God, and we align ourselves with His will.

Massage

Massage is simply the manipulation of your soft tissues by a trained individual. Research shows that massage reduces heart rate, lowers blood pressure, increases blood circulation, relaxes muscles, removes toxins from muscles, strengthens the immune system, helps relieve mental stress, reduces anxiety, improves digestion and elimination, and increases energy. That's quite a list of benefits!

In most communities, you can find trained massage therapists.

Physical exercise

You can profit from participation in hard, physical exercise such as running, tennis, basketball, rock wall climbing, and martial arts in much the same ways as you can from the more sedentary activities I have listed above.

Physical exercise is a powerful antidote to stress, acting much as antioxidants do to the toxins in our bodies. In addition, when we engage in physical activity, we must be present in the moment in order to be effective. We don't have time to think about the stresses of the day.

Physical exercise also helps to loosen and relax our muscles, it promotes blood flow, and it allows us to breathe more efficiently.

LOOKING BACK

To sum up, all of the interrelated elements of DREAM Health promote the idea of listening to your body so that you can respond to its needs. "Rest" is the second element in the DREAM acronym: diet, rest, exercise, alternative care, and motivation.

The biggest component of rest is sleep, both at night and in the form of naps. If we get enough sleep, our bodies have plenty of energy, which means we are more apt to exercise and take care of ourselves in other ways. And, of course, if we exercise more and eat better, this in turn helps us to sleep better. By now, you understand how any deficiencies or toxicities have a systemic affect on your health and well-being.

Our rest consists of more than good sound sleep; it also includes our vacation time (everything from a day off to a longer vacation) and various techniques for de-stressing our lives, such as prayer and meditation, massage, and physical exercise. These techniques counterbalance the damaging effects of stress.

As you have read this chapter, I hope you have been able to identify some new ways that you can try to get better rest every day.

☑ TO-DO LIST

☑ Practice taking a fifteen-minute rest period each day. Nap if you can.

☑ Sleep an extra hour each night this week.

☑ Look at the quality of your mattress and consider making some changes, if needed.

☑ Schedule a long weekend away from work to spend alone or with your family.

☑ Find a form of physical exercise that would be easy for you to work into your current lifestyle.

Exercise: Keeping Strong and Healthy

⁓

⁓

Your whole self—body, mind, and spirit—can only achieve whole health if you give equal attention to not only your diet and rest, but also to physical exercise. Alone, any one of these health-building components is simply inadequate; all three of them are interrelated and interdependent.

We have already explored diet and rest, and now it's time to move on to the third element of DREAM Health—exercise. We need to develop a balanced approach toward exercise, one that makes it possible for us to find the types of activities as well as the level of activity that will enable us to thrive. Our bodies were designed for sustained activity. Every cell of our bodies will benefit from an intelligent and consistent approach to keeping fit.

What is your experience of physical exercise? Does it make you remember (with dread) the musty locker room of your high school

PE class? Is your recliner or your deck chair more attractive to you than your bicycle or your kayak? What do you do after work? Vegetate in front of the TV? Watching sports, perhaps? Are you actually an avid sports fan—more faithful to purchase your season ticket than you are to play the game? Or are you out there yourself, working up a sweat?

Too many of us have been brainwashed to perceive the energy expenditure of physical exercise as an optional tool, perhaps useful to increase one's athletic performance or to lose some extra baggage in particular places, but unnecessary for the average Joe or Josephine. This way of thinking is too much like the symptom-treating mind-set of the medical establishment. In other words, too many of us feel that if parts of our bodies aren't crying out for attention, we don't need to worry about it. Or perhaps we have persuaded ourselves that what we do each day at work provides us with adequate and appropriate exercise.

Allow me to suggest a far better mind-set, one that sees good nutrition, good rest, and good exercise as a seamless whole.

CREATED FOR ACTION

Our bodies were designed to move, to be active. We have been equipped to walk and climb, lift and carry, push and persevere. Our ancestors had no problem with this concept, because their survival demanded their physical exertion. They couldn't have meat to eat without exerting themselves to go hunting or to care for their domesticated animals, not to mention the labor-intensive effort required to prepare the cut-up animal for consumption. They couldn't have vegetables and fruits to eat without gathering, gleaning, and preparing them. They couldn't even drink water without carrying it from somewhere else. At the end of each long day, they slept soundly because they were truly fatigued from their many exertions. They walked almost everywhere. Even when they rode on a donkey or in an oxcart or sailing ship, their bodies were exercised far more than ours are in the cushioned comfort of our automobiles.

Our modern twenty-first-century world denies our bodies their natural urge to *move*. Instead of finding new ways to fulfill that natural desire, we have opted to make comfort and the saving of time our primary goals. Think about it—we even drive our cars to the gym!

The fact of the matter is that when we deny our bodies the active movement that they want, we force all that energy to come out in other ways, such as mental stress and anxiety. We allow our well-designed bodies to waste away and lose effectiveness. No longer can they fight illness well. Now they are sluggish and weak.

Improving the signals

Your body is equipped with mechano-receptors that are like signal mechanisms in your joints and your muscles. The number of these signaling mechanisms increases as it approaches the spinal column and the brain. Let's say your hands and feet have hundreds of them; your elbows and knees have thousands; your shoulders and hips have hundreds of thousands; your spine has millions; your brain has multimillions of them.

These mechano-receptors signal your brain when you're moving. In your brain, this information is equated with health. When you move your muscles and joints, you enjoy improved mental acuity, decreased emotional depression, increased immune function, and an overall increased sense of well-being.

However, what if you're *not* moving very much? Then your mechano-receptors don't receive very much stimulation. Your inactivity has the opposite effect on your well-being. Your stress level rises, depression asserts itself, your immune response decreases, and toxicity builds up.

To reestablish a healthy flow of signals, we need to ask ourselves the same questions we asked about our nutrition. In this case, we ask ourselves: "Is my exercise program (or my lack of an exercise program) causing my natural healing system a deficiency? How can I provide it with sufficiency?" We also ask, "Is my exercise program (or my lack of it) causing my natural healing system to suffer from toxicity? How can I provide it with purity?"

Effects of inactivity

In one study, inactivity was shown to contribute directly to chronic disease and early death. The portion of the study group of Harvard nurses who engaged in 2.5 hours of brisk walking each week were found to have 30 percent less coronary disease and 30 percent fewer strokes than the control portion of the study group.[1] It turns out that exercise is a powerful antioxidant, which decreases factors of toxicity in the human body. Individuals who are sedentary fail to benefit from this effect, and they also suffer from increased platelet aggregation in their blood, which increases their likelihood of suffering blood clots and strokes.

The President's Council on Physical Fitness and Sports reports the following:

- A sedentary lifestyle is a major risk factor across the spectrum of preventable diseases that lower the quality of life and kill Americans.

- Physical inactivity contributes to 300,000 preventable deaths a year in the United States.

- As much as 40 percent of deaths in the United States are caused by behavior patterns that could be modified.

- Moderate daily physical activity can reduce substantially the risk of developing or dying from cardiovascular disease, type 2 diabetes, and certain cancers such as colon cancer.

- Daily physical activity helps to lower blood pressure and cholesterol, helps prevent or retard osteoporosis, and helps reduce obesity, symptoms of anxiety and depression, and symptoms of arthritis.

- Moderate physical activity includes thirty minutes of brisk walking or raking leaves, fifteen minutes of running, or forty-five minutes of playing volleyball.

- Nearly half of American adults (four out of ten) report that they are not active at all; seven out of ten are not moderately active for the recommended thirty minutes a day, five or more days a week.

- The health risk posed by inactivity is almost as high as risk factors such as cigarette smoking, high blood pressure, and high cholesterol.

- A physically active lifestyle adopted early in life may continue into adulthood. Even among children aged three and four years, those who were less active tended to remain less active than most of their peers after age three. According to a study done by the National Association of Sports and Physical Education, infants, toddlers, and preschoolers should engage in at least sixty minutes of physical activity daily and should not be sedentary for more than sixty minutes at a time, except when sleeping.

- The major barriers most people face when trying to increase physical activity are time, access to convenient facilities, and safe environments in which to be active. [2]

As a nation we are overfed and under-exercised. In 1970, American males were twenty-two pounds heavier (for height match) than in 1863. The sedentary lifestyle of so many Americans could be considered a pandemic, as could the obesity that accompanies the lack of exercise. Together, obesity and sedentary lifestyle are responsible for an enormous burden of chronic disease, impaired physical function and quality of life, and at least $90 billion in direct annual health-care costs in the United States.[3]

These health-care costs mount up quickly because of the number of life-threatening diseases that can develop because of lack of exercise. Take colon cancer, for instance. Exercise helps the human body to excrete more waste. An increase in the activity of a person's cardiovascular system increases the liquefaction of mucus, which strains through the lymph system and colon. Therefore, exercising keeps things moving well, which in turns helps to prevent colon cancer. Conversely, lack of exercise can be blamed for the high rate of colon cancer in the United States (as many as 110,000 new cases in a year, with as many as 50,000 deaths). Numerous studies have shown that among people who engage in the highest levels of exercise, the incidence of colon cancer is cut in half. Simply getting regular exercise is all it takes to protect yourself from this killer disease!

It's a pandemic of today's society— sedentary lifestyles and obesity.

The Harvard Center for Cancer Prevention reports that:

- More than half of all colorectal cancers can be prevented with lifestyle changes, such as getting exercise and eating a healthy diet.

- Many risk factors for colorectal cancer are within an individual's control and can be modified through lifestyle changes, including being physically active for at least thirty minutes per day and maintaining a healthy weight.[4]

Inactivity also contributes to the development of other forms of cancer. Studies show that obesity (most often the result of lack of exercise) accounts for 10 percent of cancer deaths among men in the United States and 15–20 percent among American women. The risks of endometrial, breast, kidney, prostate, and esophageal cancers are increased as well as the rate of colorectal cancer. According to Dr. Leslie Bernstein, professor of preventive medicine at the Keck School of Medicine, University of Southern California in Los Angeles, "The issue with obesity isn't that the gene pool has changed. The [obesity] epidemic is solely due to lifestyle changes."[5] Dr. Bernstein continues, "Exercise can play as important a role in cancer prevention as the latest screening tool or chemoprevention drug.... [For instance,] epidemiological studies strongly suggest that just a few hours each week of moderate to vigorous exercise can reduce a woman's exposure to ovarian hormones that cause breast cancer."[6]

Effects of an improved activity level

What can physical exercise do for you? For one thing, numerous studies have shown that regular, sustained cardiovascular workouts can reduce "bad cholesterol" (LDL) and increase "good cholesterol" (HDL). (LDL cholesterol is what is dumped into your arteries from the fatty foods you eat. HDL cholesterol carries extra cholesterol out of your arteries and eliminates it through the liver.)

Your personal experience will testify that when you exercise more, you can get to sleep faster and sleep more soundly. As a result, you awake more refreshed. You set a beneficial cycle into motion: feeling refreshed keeps you sharp, alert, and happy, which makes you keep up your activity level. You don't tend to overeat, you can concentrate better, you are slimmer and trimmer, you suffer from fewer ailments and injuries, and so on.

What's true for adults is certainly true for children and teenagers. Also, apparently exercise is a key for keeping your kids safer from harmful behaviors. Researchers at the University of North Carolina at Chapel Hill report that teens who participate in physical activity—especially those who are active along-side their parents—are not as likely to become involved with drinking, drugs, violence, smoking, illicit sex, and over-all delinquency as the couch-potato teens who spend a lot of time in front of the television. The researchers also assessed the self-esteem level of the teens in their study, and they determined that those who played sports with their parents had the lowest risk for poor self-esteem.[7]

> SURGEON GENERAL'S WARNING: *The Surgeon General has determined that lack of physical activity is detrimental to your health.*[8]

For both teens and adults, a higher fitness level not only improves self-esteem and reduces stress levels, but it also increases and regulates the circulation and the blood flow to the heart, increases the number of red blood cells, and increases overall blood volume. Participating in a regular exercise program results in improved cardiovascular endurance, muscle strength, and flexibility, and it assists a person in maintaining a general sense of well-being and confidence.

Researchers in Seattle studied older citizens to see what protective effects increased exercise might have against Alzheimer's and other forms of dementia.[9] Their study group consisted of 1,740 men and women over the age of sixty-five who, at the beginning of the study, scored highly on tests of mental function. Their mental and physical health was checked every two years, and they were asked to report on the number of days a week they participated in at least fifteen minutes of walking, hiking, bicycling, aerobics, weight training, and the like.

After a little over six years, 158 of the study participants had developed dementia, and calculations showed that 38 percent fewer of the participants who exercised ended up with dementia. In a summary of the study, Dr. Robert W. Griffith states, "Exercise has been proved beneficial for numerous conditions associated with aging—diabetes, cancer, heart attack, stroke, osteoporosis, and overweight. Why shouldn't it be helpful for preventing dementia too?"[10]

The greatest stress-buster

Exercise is the great stress-buster. When you get regular exercise, your stress level—from all three forms of stress: physical, emotional, and chemical—comes down. Stress is to your body what plaque is to your teeth. It's always there, unrelentingly damaging all of the systems of your body. But with exercise, you can keep much of that damage at bay.

The U.S. military has long known about the benefits of regular physical exercise and stress relief. In the *Targeting Stress Workbook: Exercise and Stress*, Major Leo Mahoney, MPT lists some of the benefits of exercise as a stress-reducing strategy:[11]

1. Regular exercise helps one to feel in control. This sense of control over the body may translate to an improved sense of control over other aspects of life, a key defense against stress.

2. Exercise promotes well-being and relaxation. Regular exercisers demonstrate higher levels of self-esteem and confidence and maintain a sense of self-discipline. The individual acts upon the belief, "I am in charge of myself and can improve my health and fitness."

3. Moderate physical activity is a natural, physiological outlet for a body in the "fight or flight" state of arousal

frequently associated with stress. It cleanses the body of adrenaline, can lower the blood pressure, and relaxes tight muscles.

4. Exercise produces neurotransmitters called endorphins in the brain. These are the body's own natural tranquilizers. Endorphins can make one feel calm and relaxed during and for up to three hours after moderate physical activity. This elevation in mood has been referred to as the runners' high but is also experienced by those involved in other forms of exercise.

5. Exercise can cause many people who are physically active to give up unhealthy and stressful habits that interfere with exercise [and health]. Smokers may cut down or quit....Others may eat more nutritiously to improve performance. The chronically busy individual may "work in" a workout to increase energy, alertness and productivity.

Exercise is an inexpensive and achievable tool for achieving total health, and it comes with extra benefits. Leo Mahoney also said, "The old adages 'run for your life' and 'burn off some steam' merit serious consideration. It is truly possible to walk, bike, run, lift, and stretch your way to a happier, less stressful lifestyle."[12]

Regular exercise, according the *Annals of Behavioral Medicine*, helped 135 undergraduate university students cope with the stress they experienced, which included everything from major life events to having minor car trouble.[13] The key to better coping was their level of leisure physical activity. The students whose lifestyles included more activity had less anxiety and fewer physical complaints than the students who were inactive. Well-maintained fitness seemed to buffer the effects of their normal life stress load.

People who undertake regular exercise experience greater over-all happiness, more satisfaction in life, and decreased depression. The decrease in depression is most likely the result of the release of serotonin, norepinephrine, and dopamine, which are neurotransmitters that act as natural antidepressants. Abundant research points to a link between a deficiency of these neurotransmitters and depression, anxiety, impulsivity, aggression, and increased appetite.

Psychiatric researchers from Boston University School of Medicine report:

> Millions of Americans suffer from clinical depression each year. Most depressed patients first seek treatment from their primary care providers. Generally, depressed patients treated in primary care settings receive pharmacologic therapy alone. There is evidence to suggest that the addition of cognitive-behavioral therapies, *specifically exercise,* can improve treatment outcomes for many patients. *Exercise is a behavioral intervention that has shown great promise in alleviating symptoms of depression.*[14]

High cost of the American sedentary lifestyle

With obesity and sedentary lifestyles causing a staggering $90 billion of health-care expenses annually, how does that cost break down?

Osteoporosis, which is a major problem of older women, incurs one set of cost factors that can be traced directly to lack of exercise. Loss of bone density is 100 percent preventable with the right combination of nutrition and fitness. Note—I said "combination." You can eat all the right foods and take all the right supplements and still suffer from osteoporosis. Strong bones are not created unless the body is under the regular, physical stress of exercise. A sedentary lifestyle is a virtual guarantee of osteoporosis, especially in postmenopausal women, and osteoporosis puts older people at great risk for fractures, many of which prove to be fatal. Estimates of low bone density in women over the age of fifty range from 50 percent to 68 percent. The cost of treating fractures from osteoporosis exceeds \$14 billion per year (that's about \$38 million per *day*)[15]—all for a deficiency that could be easily prevented by informed nutritional choices, balanced and enhanced by regular exercise.

WHAT'S *YOUR* EXCUSE?

Most people say that the reason they don't get enough exercise is because they lack:

1. Time
2. Energy

Is this true for you as well?

Would it help you to hear that one of the first rewards of an exercise program is more energy? And with a higher energy level, often your daily activities take less time, which frees up more time for exercise. So, ironically, it is important to pursue a fitness program even if you don't feel you have enough time and energy to do so.

Perhaps part of our problem is the human tendency to think, *It won't happen to me.* Each of us feels that we will be the exception to the rule. "*I* can go ahead and eat fast food and be a couch potato. It's been OK so far. Nothing has killed me yet."

Or we procrastinate: "I'll wait until the kids are all in school." "I'll wait until this crazy project at work is finished." "I'll wait until summer." "I'll start next week." The whole excuse-making exercise gives us a false sense of security. Meanwhile, our bodies are registering the lack of exercise, whether we can see the warning signs or not.

We need to get motivated to change. We need to remember that "life is motion." We need to be reminded of these sobering words:

You only receive one body for your entire lifetime. If you only had one house, one car, and one set of clothes in this lifetime, how would you maintain them? What kind of care would you offer them to ensure longevity and durability? The sad truth is that often we spend more on our cars, homes, and clothes than we do on taking care of the body that God has given us. Of course, we spend thousands of dollars on medical bills once we have become ill. It would seem more reasonable to spend some of those dollars on maintenance to avoid the high cost of illness.[16]

Must you exercise for the prescribed thirty minutes daily? Is that feasible? Perhaps you truly do not have the time for that. But *any amount* of intentional exercise will help your health. Research indicates that it takes only a relatively short, low-impact workout to increase one's overall fitness level.

Try exercising for only ten minutes at a time, and work up to three times a day, a total of thirty minutes a day. Or try simply working more activity into your daily routine. Take the stairs instead of the elevator; mow your lawn, rake your leaves, weed your flowerbed; park farther away from your destination so you have to walk; get off the bus a few blocks before your regular stop so you can walk the rest of the way.

In a report titled "Physical Activity and Health," published on the Web site for the National Center for Chronic Disease Prevention and Health Promotion, the United States Surgeon General laments:

> Despite common knowledge that exercise is healthful, more than 60 percent of American adults are not regularly active, and 25 percent of the adult population is not active at all. Moreover, although many people have enthusiastically embarked on vigorous exercise programs at one time or another, most do not sustain their participation. Clearly, the processes of developing and maintaining

healthier habits are as important to study as the health effects of these habits.[17]

Our motivation needs as much attention as does our active physical exercise. Regular activity results in something we call "fitness," but our idea of what fitness means can discourage us from the outset. Consider the word *fitness*. Does the word make you think of having a lean, muscular body, one that is in top shape for strenuous activities such as hiking long distances, swimming competitively, running in races, or skiing the difficult slopes? If that's all that it means, most of us do not have the time or desire to become a model of fitness.

We spend the first half of our lives giving up our health to get money. Then we spend the second half of our lives giving up our money to try to regain our health.

However, nearly all of us can reach for a level of fitness that allows for good health and the ability to pursue our life goals. Sports physiologists usually define fitness as (1) having adequate muscular strength and endurance to accomplish one's individual goals; (2) having reasonable joint flexibility; (3) having an efficient cardiovascular system; and (4) having a body composition that falls within the normal range of body weight and percent of body fat.[18]

To be fit, we must engage regularly in activities that challenge our minds and bodies to perform beyond what is required by a couch-potato lifestyle. If our quest for fitness is pursued sporadically, the beneficial effects will be quickly lost.

Personally, I would like to be different from the bulk of the population—I would like to be fit and healthy. Wouldn't you like to join me? Let's get motivated. Let's make one of the most sensible commitments we ever made—let's get more physical exercise on a regular, sustainable basis.

Our fitness programs will fall into two major categories: *aerobic training*, which improves endurance and increases the body's ability to utilize oxygen, and *anaerobic training*, which enhances the size and strength of particular muscles and body regions.

AEROBIC EXERCISE

Aerobic exercise causes a person to breathe harder and to therefore sustain an elevated heart rate over an extended period of time. It also burns fat, although it takes about twenty minutes of sustained aerobic exercise before the body starts to use its stored fat as fuel. Aerobic exercise is crucial for cardiovascular health, weight loss, and body-shaping.

The main objective of aerobic exercise is to increase the maximum amount of oxygen that the body can process within a given time. Regular aerobic exercise raises the body's metabolism so that the body burns more calories all the time, even when it is at rest.

Your daily minimum of thirty minutes of exercise should consist of aerobic types of activity. These would include jogging, swimming laps, hiking and walking, cross-country skiing, martial arts, rope-skipping, stair-climbing, bicycling, and active sports such as hockey, basketball, and tennis.

Heart rate

Before you begin an aerobic exercise program, you might want to determine your target heart rate range. Your target heart rate is the pulse rate that you are working toward. You want to exercise safely, not overtaxing your heart or the rest of your body, but you also want to receive the maximum cardiovascular benefits of your workout.

Your age and your general health condition will determine your target heart rate. The easiest way to calculate it is to subtract your age from 220. The result is your maximum heart rate (the number of pulse beats per minute). To check your heart rate, place your fingers just under your jaw line under your ear. Count your heartbeats for six seconds and multiply the number of beats by ten.

If you are just beginning an exercise program, you should strive to achieve 60–75 percent of your maximum heart rate. If you have been exercising for some time, you can safely exercise up to about 85 percent of your maximum heart rate. You can adjust the level of your workout as needed to adjust to your target heart rate range.

STEPS OF AN AEROBIC WORKOUT

Each of your workout sessions should include the following steps:

1. **Warm-up** (five minutes). Warming up is easy to do; it is simply doing your chosen activity, such as walking, at a slower pace. Warming up will loosen up your muscles and prepare your body for exercise.

2. **Pre-exercise stretching.** Stretching improves flexibility, decreases muscle soreness, and aids in relaxation.[19]

3. **Physical activity** (five to ten minutes at first, gradually increasing to thirty to forty-five minutes). During this portion of activity, strive to work within your target heart rate range.

4. **Cool-down** (five minutes). Your cool-down period allows your heart rate, breathing, and blood pressure to return to normal. As with the warm-up step, simply decrease your activity to a slower pace. Check your pulse rate—your pulse level should be down to at least 100 beats per minute before you stop moving and begin the stretching phase.

5. **Post-exercise stretching** (five to ten minutes). It is important to stretch both before and after exercising. Hold each stretch for twenty to thirty seconds, without bouncing.

Walking

Of all the types of aerobic activity, walking is the easiest. It is excellent exercise for a person of either gender in any age group, and it requires no equipment except a pair of comfortable walking shoes. You can walk anywhere—in your neighborhood, at the mall, in your office building.

Walking produces less stress on your joints than most other forms of aerobic exercise. This makes it ideal as a basic activity throughout one's life, and also an effective starting place for those who are just beginning a fitness program. You can start out with five or ten minutes a day and slowly work your way up to thirty minutes or more, even if you are so busy that it must be split into ten-minute chunks. You don't have to walk all by yourself. You can plan to walk daily with your spouse or child or a friend, or you can take your dog for a brisk stroll.

ANAEROBIC EXERCISE

Anaerobic exercise is activity such as resistance training, which uses muscles at high intensity for a short period of time. Anaerobic exercise increases muscle strength and flexibility. It includes push-ups and pull-ups, stomach crunches, sprinting, and resistance or strength training.

Resistance training

Resistance or strength training involves the use of some form of resistance such as free weights or nautilus equipment to strengthen, tone, and sometimes build the size of various muscles groups.

As it builds muscle strength, resistance training also reduces stress levels and builds bone density. It is not only for bodybuilders who want to increase their muscle size, but also for anyone who wants to keep his body strong, healthy, and fit. Besides building strength, resistance training provides a person with a cardiovascular workout; if the rest time between sets of exercises is minimized, a person can maintain a moderate heart rate throughout the entire workout. This strengthens the most important muscle in your body—your heart.

Strength training

Strength training can be accomplished by various means. To start, you could purchase some small ankle or arm weights and wear them while walking around your house. Or lift small weights while watching television, during the commercial breaks.

Another good way to begin strength training is isometrics—pushing against an immovable object. Isometric training can include push-ups, pull-ups, chin-ups, and sit-ups. Whenever you are flexing or applying force against something—including your own body, such as when you press one palm against the other—you are doing isometrics. The important action is muscle contraction—pushing, pressing, pulling—which uses minimal movement but builds your muscles. Pulling in the muscles of your abdomen is an isometric exercise. So is the Kegel exercise, a contraction of the vaginal muscle that most women are taught during and after pregnancy and childbirth.

You can do isometric exercises almost anywhere and anytime. You can start by holding each muscle contraction for five seconds, then releasing it. You can work up to ten or fifteen seconds per contraction, and do them in sets of ten. Your "equipment" is minimal and easy to find. For example, you can stand in a doorway and, holding your hands thigh-high, press the backs of your hands outward against the sides of the door frame as hard as you can. Hold and release, then repeat. Or, if you are tall enough, stand in a doorway and press one hand at a time against the top of the door frame. Then you can bend your elbows and press your palms outward against the door frame at chest level. Next, you can move over to the wall and do a series of "standing push-ups" against it.

KEEPING MOTIVATED

The kinds of exercises you choose will depend upon your physical abilities, your other commitments, and your preferences. Even if you choose an activity that you enjoy, it can be hard to maintain a regular exercise schedule. Perhaps you could work out with a friend or with your spouse and keep each other motivated.

Health clubs and some gyms will design resistance- and strength-training programs to match your personal goals, and some health club plans include the services of a personal trainer. A personal trainer can design a plan that works for you and help to keep you motivated over an extended period of time.

The best systems for alternative care operate out of a "whole-earth" wholeness paradigm. They stand in stark contrast to those systems that concentrate only on one limited, "flat-earth" viewpoint for treating specific symptoms of sickness.

Remember to start slow and work up to your goals. Don't fall into the very common mistake of planning an over-ambitious exercise regimen that is unrealistic over the long haul. That will be a formula for defeat, because you will likely quit before you see the many benefits of consistent, varied exercise. Besides, if you gradually increase both the length and the intensity of your physical activity, your body will not be thrown into survival mode, which tends to suppress your immune system instead of strengthening it.

Remember also to include some variety in your exercise plan. You don't want to get bored with it, and you don't want to develop one part of your body while neglecting another. Your body, which carries the genetic capability for a life of hunting and gathering and other life-sustaining activity, requires an ebbing and flowing of exertion and a variety of health-promoting stresses.

Remember also to allow for rest times for the various parts of your body that are being exercised. You could try alternating days of heart-pumping aerobic exercise and strength-building anaerobic resistance training. Your body will thank you, and you will be rewarded with the health you desire.

HOW MANY CALORIES DOES IT BURN?

A pound is the equivalent of approximately 3,500 calories. In order to lose one pound a week, you need to eliminate approximately 500 calories a day through diet or exercise or a combination of both. How much exercise does it take to burn off that 500 calories? Here is a list of activities with the average calories burned per *minute*:

- 2.0 to 2.5—standing, sleeping, sitting
- 2.5 to 4.0—walking slowly (2 miles/hour), bicycling slowly (5 miles/hour)
- 4.0 to 5.0—walking or bicycling medium-fast (3 miles/hour and 6 miles/hour), playing badminton, doing housework
- 5.0 to 6.0—walking fast (4 miles/hour), playing doubles tennis, dancing, raking leaves, doing calisthenics
- 6.0 to 7.0—ice- or inline-skating, bicycling fast (10 miles/hour)

- 7.0 to 8.0—walking briskly (5 miles/hour), downhill skiing, playing singles tennis, water-skiing

- 8.0 to 10.0—playing basketball, mountain-climbing, jogging slowly (5 miles/hour), bicycling competitively (12 miles/hour)

- 10.0 to 11.0—jogging quickly (6 miles/hour), cross-country skiing, playing racquetball or handball

- 12.0—swimming laps

LOOKING BACK

An exercise plan, combined with a nutritious and moderate eating plan and a sensible amount of daily rest, creates optimal health. Most advisors, including the United States Surgeon General and the American College of Sports Medicine, recommend that every American should accumulate thirty minutes or more of daily, moderate-intensity physical exercise. One simple way to meet this standard would be to incorporate a brisk two-mile walk into your typical day. For an adult, this should be enough to expend 200 calories. If you cannot walk two miles a day, in all likelihood, you are sitting too much. For more complete exercise guidelines, go to my Web site, www .DREAMHealth.com.

Train yourself to have a healthy aversion to a sedentary lifestyle and its accompanying health problems. Your body thrives on activity and motion. Stand up—right now—and move!

☑ TO-DO LIST

☑ Prior to beginning a fitness routine, check with your health-care provider. Start slow and progress gradually.

☑ Pick an aerobic activity that you enjoy, and spend at least twenty to thirty minutes, three times a week, on that activity.

☑ Pick a resistance-training activity, and work it into your schedule twice a week.

☑ Include warm-up and cool-down times in your activities.

☑ Decide what will keep you motivated, such as planning to work out with a friend, and make sure that continued motivation is one of your goals.

Alternative Care: Your Best Health Insurance

⁓

*Dear friend, I pray that you may enjoy good health and that all may
go well with you, even as your soul is getting along well.*

—3 JOHN 2

⁓

I have included alternative care as the fourth of the five integral components of DREAM Health (the *A*) because I am convinced that none of us will get an *A* in our health without the assistance of qualified alternative care givers. Without their help, your body's self-healing process will probably get off track at some point, but *with* their beneficial services, you can keep yourself healthy and strong for the rest of your life.

What do I mean by "alternative care"? As defined by the National Library of Medicine, alternative medical care is, broadly speaking, "Any of various systems of healing or treating disease that are not included in the traditional curricula taught in medical schools of the United States and Britain."[1] Alternative care includes a long list of disciplines, and you can read about some of them by visiting the Web site of the National Center for Complementary and Alternative

Medicine (http://nccam.nih.gov), which is part of the National Institutes of Health. NCCAM collects and disseminates information about a wide variety of types of *alternative care* (care that is used instead of conventional medical care) or *complementary care* (care that is used alongside selected methods of conventional medical care), including chiropractic care, massage therapy, acupuncture, dietary supplementation, and much more.

WHY IS THIS CONSIDERED "ALTERNATIVE"?

For most of human history, what we now call alternative care actually dominated the health-care landscape. Folk medicine, herbal medicine, and many culturally traditional methods of healing were the only methods available. But at the turn of the twentieth century, there was a great shift. Many people date it to 1901, when philanthropist John D. Rockefeller founded the Rockefeller Institute for Medical Research in New York City, and also to 1913, when he founded the Rockefeller Foundation, the work of which was focused largely on public health and medical training and which endowed now-prestigious medical institutions, including Johns Hopkins School of Hygiene and Public Health. With Rockefeller funding, medical research and development really took off to become the mammoth, research-based industry that it is now.

Today, about one hundred years later, what used to be considered traditional, conventional medicine is termed "alternative," while the reverse is true of the medical care that studies and treats symptoms of disease—what we practitioners of alternative medicine call "allopathic" medicine. (*Allopath—Allos* means "opposite" and *path* means "disease." Allopathic medicine aims to relieve the symptoms of disease, and it relies almost exclusively on pharmaceutical drugs and invasive surgeries to obtain the desired results. Alternative medicine does not.)

Ironically and alarmingly, despite the fact that most of us put our faith and trust in allopathic medicine, the overall population is now *less* healthy than ever, and our health care is costing us more money. As people realize what is happening, more and more of them are turning to alternative care, especially because it offers so many low-risk and effective choices for proactive and preventive care of one's personal health. Such people believe that it is a wise move to choose the most conservative, least invasive methods first, only falling back on the riskier alternatives in times of crisis.

Whole earth or flat earth?

As I have already mentioned, I prefer to use the words *holistic* or *wholeness* when referring to alternative care. This goes along with my view that only within these wellness-promoting modalities do we find "whole-earth" care.

Is the earth flat, as it appears to be when you look out from your bedroom window? Or is it round, as seen only from a superior perspective? Christopher Columbus gave us the answer to that question. The whole earth is a sphere, not a pancake. Correspondingly, the best systems for alternative care operate out of a "whole-earth" wholeness paradigm. They stand in stark contrast to those systems that concentrate only on one limited, "flat-earth" viewpoint for treating specific symptoms of sickness.

A holistic philosophy approaches health and wellness by recognizing the self-healing abilities of the human body and by considering the whole person rather than merely the physical problems that currently afflict the person. While allopathic medicine treats the symptoms of an illness with drugs, alternative care therapies look to the cause of the symptoms. They help to strengthen the human body's natural process of healing itself, thus eliminating the symptoms of ill health.

Least invasive, least risky

Alternative care professionals who hold a whole-earth viewpoint facilitate healing. They do not provide merely a temporary, palliative cure. A holistic philosophy uses the least invasive tools first, such as giving you advice about changing your diet or your posture, and it only resorts to invasive methods after first giving you a chance to get healthy on your own.

If you had a garden and wanted to get rid of a big weed growing in the middle of your garden, you wouldn't start by bringing the most invasive weed-pulling tool, a bulldozer, would you? You would use the least invasive method first—a hoe or a trowel. It's the same with alternative care. You start simple and keep the whole person in mind.

It's not that any one approach to alternative care can provide for all of your health needs. (You won't go to your acupuncturist to be fitted for bifocals.) And it's not the case that everybody who falls under the umbrella of alternative care is operating out of the wholeness mentality. But if you look for alternative care specialists whose goal is to support your health and the well-being of your whole body, mind, and spirit, I believe that you will be better off for it.

Naturally, because I am a chiropractor myself, I believe that chiropractic is by far the largest example of successful alternative care and that it possesses the most holistic viewpoint.

Greater benefit

You can seek your health-care providers with your eyes open, informed about what you really want out of the relationship. Look for someone who combines all of the qualities you are looking for. Unless you live in a remote location, you undoubtedly have many choices, and you can change your mind if you want to. Consult your friends or other health-care providers to recommend their preferred practice. Visit Web sites such as http://www.chiropractic.org (the

International Chiropractic Association) to find contact information for the alternative care treatment centers near you. Remember, you are your own primary care doctor, and you must take control of your own health.

When you are searching for a good alternative care provider, you can make a first appointment for a consultation, in which you can essentially interview the potential alternative care provider before you submit to treatments. Ask whatever questions you want. A trustworthy professional will confidently answer your questions to your satisfaction.

Ask the candidate, "What are your clinical goals for me?" If the answer is, "Providing you with relief from your symptoms of disease," that person is following an allopathic model of medical care. If the reply is, "Reducing your symptoms of disease through natural cures," that person too is following an allopathic model, albeit by less risky, more natural means. But if the answer to your question is, "Moving you toward wholeness in your mind, body, and spirit," and especially if they add "through Christ," then most likely you are in the right place.

You may want to be careful of practitioners who practice "natural" medicine but whose philosophy is based in religions or beliefs that denigrate the true God who created you and in whom you trust. With any form of alternative medicine, you should watch for metaphysical/New Age language ("positive and negative energies," "the god within you," and so on) and projection (being instructed to leave your body). Always compare the philosophies being presented to the truth of the Bible.

If at any point you feel uncomfortable with instructions or language used by a practitioner, move on to someone else. But don't give up! There are many modern professionals who offer these therapies without any spiritual context at all. You can also find Christian practitioners who replace other religious influences with godly, biblical principles so that Christians can reap the physical and mental benefits of various forms of alternative care without worrying about the "spiritual side effects."

I (along with a growing army of others) also believe that physical *touch* is a key component of health. Alternative care providers, without any high-tech medical machinery and rooms full of gadgets, accomplish as much as (or more than) their counterparts in our nation's medical centers. By personality, disposition, and training, alternative care providers convey compassionate warmth when they meet with a patient. They are knowledgeable and capable, but they haven't had to become glorified technicians, which is what too much of the medical establishment has been required to become. The gentle, caring, physical touch of alternative care is good for you!

Just say no to drugs

Once you have decided that you don't want to travel the drug route over and over, you'll need to ask questions about the relative effectiveness of alternative forms of treatment, not to mention the less likely but nevertheless possible side effects of alternative therapies.

Here is an interesting bit of information: the Greek word *pharmakeia,* from which our word *pharmaceuticals* (i.e., prescription drugs) is derived, is used in the Bible; it is translated into English as "witchcraft."[2] (See Galatians 5:20.) This isn't to say that all prescription drugs are evil like witchcraft, but it does serve as a caution. Before you put your unquestioning faith in drugs—or in the latest natural herbal discovery—you need to decide whether the effects of that substance will carry an influence that is more powerful than you expected.

WHO SEEKS ALTERNATIVE CARE?

More and more people are choosing to explore alternative care for their health and wellness needs.

Health psychologist John Astin completed a study about the most popular types of alternative care and the most frequently treated health problems. He found that "forty percent of respondents reported using some form of alternative health care during the past year. The top four treatment categories were chiropractic (15.7 percent), lifestyle diet (8 percent), exercise/movement (7.2 percent), and relaxation (6.9 percent). The most frequently cited health problems treated with alternative therapies were chronic pain (37 percent), anxiety, chronic fatigue syndrome and 'other health condition' (31 percent each), sprains/muscle strains (26 percent), addictive problems and arthritis (both 25 percent) and headaches (24 percent)."[3]

In general, Astin's survey found that those who prefer alternative or complementary health therapies "tend to hold a philosophical orientation toward health that can be described as holistic and are more likely than others to have had some type of transformational experience that changed their world view in a significant way." The philosophy of people who choose alternative care includes recognizing "the importance of mind and spirit as well as body and health."[4]

In a now famous 1993 article, the *New England Journal of Medicine* published the results of a survey in what it called "unconventional medicine":

> The report detailed the findings of a 1990 survey of health-care utilization in the United States, suggesting that more than 30 percent of American adults availed themselves of at least one form of alternative therapy that year, paying an estimated 425 million visits

to providers of such treatments—about 40 million more than the number made to primary care physicians! The tab for this care was nearly $14 billion, of which more than $10 billion was not covered by insurance and thus was paid out of pocket.

The survey indicated that unconventional therapies were used mostly for chronic rather than life-threatening conditions.[5]

This and many other surveys show that the use of alternative care is widely spread among all social and demographic groups and that its use is increasing steadily.

In an editorial in the *Journal of the American Medical Association*, Wayne B. Jonas states, "Alternative medicine is here to stay" because its use "reflects changing needs and values in modern society." These changes were summarized as "a rise in prevalence of chronic disease, an increase in public access to worldwide health information, reduced tolerance for paternalism, an increased sense of entitlement to a quality of life, declining faith that scientific breakthroughs will have relevance for the personal treatment of disease, and increased interest in spiritualism. In addition, concern about the adverse effects and escalating costs of conventional health care are fueling the search for alternative approaches to the prevention and management of illness."[6]

What are some of the primary types of alternative care?

CHIROPRACTIC CARE

I first sought chiropractic care when I was fifteen years old. I had suffered a sports injury in my lower back, and I had been subject to migraine headaches. I was also having trouble with bed-wetting. The back pain, the migraines, and the bed-wetting all vanished after I began receiving chiropractic care.

Even though my parents' HMO did not recommend chiropractic care, it only took one visit to begin to appreciate the difference between the personal touch of chiropractic care and the traditional (insurance-subsidized) health-care clinic that I had visited previously. At the clinic, I would see a different person every time I went in, usually a physician's assistant or a nurse. It seemed that the person would take all of five minutes to evaluate my problem, prescribe a drug, and send me on my way. The chiropractor took time to develop a health-care plan for me and educate me about how to maintain my health.

I learned that the main focus of chiropractic care is the expression of each person's God-given healing potential, and that chiropractic care was the third-largest medical field after traditional medicine and dentistry, licensed in all fifty states of the United States.

As a result of my experience and what I learned, I decided early in life that I wanted to become a licensed chiropractor myself. Now, as part of my own DREAM Health lifestyle, I continue to have my own nervous system checked weekly, before any interference, misalignment, or subluxation can occur. This enables me to maintain optimum health.

> *Chiropractic care today is where dentistry was fifty years ago.*

The premise of chiropractic care

The premise of chiropractic care is based on the fact that the human brain, via the human nervous system, communicates with every cell in the body regarding its ongoing functioning. The spinal cord connects the brain with all of the branches that go out to every part of the body. In other words, the nervous system is the highway of information and internal healing. Each time you feel a touch on a part of your body, the nerve highway of information is activated.

The spinal cord is housed in the vertebral column: seven cervical vertebrae (neck region), twelve thoracic vertebrae (upper back region), five lumbar vertebrae (lower back region), and five sacral vertebrae (below the lower back). This column of vertebrae is like a suit of armor around the spinal cord; it protects it and allows it to convey signals back and forth between the brain and the parts of the body. But if stresses cause the vertebrae to become misaligned in any way, the resulting nerve pressure and inflammation choke off the free transmission of signals and, as a result, the body's own internal healing system.

The basis of chiropractic care is to perform adjustments on the spine in order to alleviate the pressure on nerves, rehabilitate and reconstruct the damage the nerves have suffered, and allow the body's natural healing power to restore balance and health to the person. If the damage is not addressed, the blockage can cause, first, dis-ease, which is the lack of ease or free function in the body, followed by the development of a diagnosable disease or illness.

A key component of chiropractic philosophy is that the human body is always regenerating and replacing itself. Did you know that every seven years, every cell of your body does this? The turnover is total, assuming that your body is healthy and strong. Chiropractic care is an ideal way to achieve optimal health and regenerative strength within your body.

Now, no one can maintain the necessary balance and alignment within the body if that person only gets chiropractic attention when the symptoms of some ailment manifest themselves. By then, it's too late to recover health quickly, because the underlying problem has been developing for a long, long time. That is why I believe so strongly in alternative care. You need to keep your immune system and all your other bodily functions tuned up so that you won't ever develop a disease in the first place. It's as simple as that.

Chiropractic care today is where dentistry was fifty years ago. At that time, people went to their dentists only when they had a problem or a symptom. Then dentists began to offer annual dental hygiene and X-rays and other services to catch developing problems early and head them off before they could become too major to fix. Now most people (with the blessing of their dental insurance providers) visit the dentist once or twice a year just for a dental health checkup. In the same way, regular visits to your chiropractor will keep your nervous system free of interference and your body healthy and whole.

Testimonials

As a chiropractic physician, I have seen tens of thousands of patients. The ones who have continued to receive chiropractic care have reaped superior health benefits. Here are several testimonials from my files:

I had headaches, neck pain, low energy, low back stiffness.

Results after chiropractic care: Now I have no more headaches! I feel my body healing itself. I no longer have neck pain while I'm driving. I'm on the road a lot, so that is a huge plus. Another bonus of chiropractic care is I no longer have indigestion. I didn't even know that chiropractic care would take care of my indigestion, but it has.

—JACK

In 1994, I injured my back while snowboarding, which ultimately became a ten-year struggle with chronic sciatica. I tried every conventional treatment and medication available with no success. My condition impacted my active lifestyle, because I was no longer able to maintain the level of activity I enjoyed and desired without triggering a major debilitating flare-up. In August of 2003, I decided to explore chiropractic care after hearing it was used to treat sciatica successfully.

Results after chiropractic care: After one year of chiropractic care, my sciatica has gradually improved. I have been pain-free for the longest stretch of time since my injury, all the while being physically active. I have been able to run again, which I never thought possible before chiropractic care!

—TREY

I have fibromyalgia, a very painful disease. I am one of the few who cannot be helped by medication. I was always looking for ways to stop the pain.

Results after chiropractic care: The first two treatments started flares, but they lasted days instead of weeks. The third treatment was pain-free! I am now in my second month of three visits a week, and the foot that I used to have to pull in when I walked has quit splaying out.

—EDWINA

These testimonials speak for themselves. Chiropractic care works, and should be at the top of everyone's list of alternative care preferences.

You can find a licensed chiropractor in your local area by searching on the Web site of the International Chiropractors Association (http://www.chiropractic.org/doctorfinder).

MASSAGE THERAPY

After chiropractic care, the most popular type of alternative care is massage therapy. The National Center for Complementary and Alternative Medicine states that "surveys of the U.S. population suggest that between 3 percent and 16 percent of adults receive chiropractic manipulation in a given year, while between 2 percent and 14 percent receive some form of massage therapy."[7] Almost every community has at least one licensed chiropractor and one certified massage therapist. I personally visit a massage therapist on a monthly basis as a form of maintenance care.

Massage therapists believe that muscle tissues are moldable, moveable, and stretchable, and that by loosening and lengthening those muscles, unwanted pressures on a person's body and nervous system are released. When you receive a good massage, it breaks up your stress, relaxes you, and causes toxins to be processed out of your body. It increases blood flow, reduces muscle spasticity, and increases lymphatic flow. Massage therapy can trigger the release of endorphins, which are the body's natural painkillers, and it can also improve mobility and flexibility. Massage therapy is an excellent complementary therapy with other types of alternative care.

Don't be confused by the various types of massage therapy. Here are the primary ones:

Swedish (or spa) massage

Five primary motions or strokes characterize traditional Swedish massage, and most Swedish massage therapists use variations on these.[8] The strokes are called: (1) *Effleurage*—long gliding strokes performed with a whole hand or with thumb pads only, often toward the heart to aid blood and lymphatic flow. (2) *Petrissage*—gentle lifting of muscles away from bones, followed by rolling and squeezing with gentle pressure. The kneading motion enhances deeper circulation and purports to clear out toxins in soft muscle and nerve tissue. (3) *Friction*—deep, circular or crosswise movements made with thumb pads or sensitive fingertips to tissues near joints and other bony areas; this stroke is believed to break down knots of muscle fibers. (4) *Tapotement*—repetitive striking or tapping movements done with the edge of the hand, tips of the fingers, or closed fist, meant to invigorate the muscles. (5) *Vibration, shaking*—rapid, controlled shaking that lasts a few seconds at a time, meant to boost circulation and increase the muscles' ability to contract.[9]

Rolfing

Rolfing is named after its founder, Dr. Ida P. Rolf, who in 1971 founded the Rolf Institute. Dr. Rolf developed Rolfing principles through her study of yoga, osteopathy, and homeopathy. Rolfers are trained to perform a kind of soft tissue manipulation that is like massage, but with an emphasis on educating the recipient to be aware of whatever may be interfering with their alignment with the earth's gravitational field.

Hellerwork

Named for its founder, Joseph Heller, Hellerwork is a deep tissue manipulation method that uses techniques similar to Rolfing. Hellerwork looks at body alignment, muscular tension, and emotional issues to provide recipients with a sense of ease and balance between their body, mind, and spirit.

Alexander Technique

"The Alexander Technique is not so much something you learn as something you unlearn"—so begins an article about the method of learning how to move your body into more ideal positions.[10] "It is a method of releasing unwanted muscular tension throughout your body which has accumulated over many years of stressful living. This excess tension often starts in childhood and, if left unchecked, can give rise in later life to common ailments....The Alexander Technique can help us to become aware of balance, posture and coordination while performing everyday actions."[11]

To find a certified massage therapist near you, visit one or more of the following Web sites:

- http://www.amtamassage.org/findamassage/locator.htm
- http://www.massagetherapy.com/find/index.php
- http://www.qwl.com/mtwc/mts

ACUPUNCTURE

Acupuncture is the ancient Chinese method of restoring the balance between the physical, emotional, and spiritual aspects of the patient. In the United States, acupuncture incorporates traditions from Japan, Korea, and other countries as well as China. It became better known in the United States in 1971, when *New York Times* reporter James Reston wrote about how doctors in China used needles to ease his pain after surgery. According to the 2002 National Health Interview Survey—the largest and most comprehensive survey of complementary and alternative medicine used by American adults to date—an estimated 8.2 million American adults have tried acupuncture.[12]

Acupuncturists insert very thin needles made of solid metal into specific anatomical points on the patient's skin to stimulate energy flow and remove blockages in order to facilitate the release of the body's own healing power. The needles are then manipulated by hand or by electrical stimulation to increase brain activity, boost the immune system, and provide relief from pain by releasing endorphins.

The World Health Organization, cognizant of the variety of traditional medical practices that flourish in the many countries of the world, issued this statement about acupuncture: "Scientific evidence from randomized clinical trials is…strong for many uses of acupuncture.…Acupuncture has been proven effective in relieving postoperative pain, nausea during pregnancy, nausea and vomiting resulting from chemotherapy, and dental pain with extremely low side effects. It can also alleviate anxiety, panic disorders and insomnia."[13]

Acupuncture is a widely accepted method of alternative care. To find an acupuncturist in your local area, you can search by means of the search function on the following Web sites:

- http://www.medicalacupuncture.org/findadoc/index
  .html
- http://www.acufinder.com
- http://www.aaom.org/45000.asp
- http://dol.jkmcomm.com/acupuncture/default.asp
- http://www.tai.edu/fp.html

ACUPRESSURE

Acupressure is described as acupuncture without needles. Based on the principles of acupuncture, acupressure involves the use of finger pressure on specific points on the body to release blocked energy so that it can flow. Acupressure stimulates and activates the body's ability to fight illness. It also helps to restore normal blood flow to the organs, revitalize the nervous system, regulate the secretions of the endocrine glands, activate the functions of internal organs, and strengthen the immune system's response.

To find a practitioner of acupressure, go to one of the following Web sites:

- http://www.acupressure.com/referral.htm
- http://www.aobta.org/find_a_member.php
- http://www.nccaom.org/find.htm

NATUROPATHY

Naturopathy, which includes many disciplines of alternative medicine such as chiropractic care, originated in Germany. Naturopathy (the word means "nature disease") views disease as an interference with the processes by which the human body can heal itself naturally, and it emphasizes the restoration of health as well as treatment of disease symptoms.

The six principles that undergird naturopathy as it is practiced in the United States are not entirely unique to naturopathy. They are:

1. The healing power of nature
2. Identification and treatment of the cause of disease
3. The concept of "first do no harm"
4. The doctor as teacher
5. Treatment of the whole person
6. Prevention[14]

Naturopathy involves diet modification and nutritional supplements, herbal medicine, acupuncture and Chinese medicine, hydrotherapy, massage and joint manipulation, and lifestyle counseling. Treatment protocols combine what the practitioner deems to be the most suitable therapies for the individual patient.[15]

HYDROTHERAPY

Hydrotherapy, as the name implies, involves water. Hydrotherapy includes saunas, baths, compresses, whirlpools, and even drinking water. Water, in all of its forms—hot or cold liquid, steam, ice—is used in hydrotherapy both inside the body and externally to cleanse and revitalize a person.

Hydrotherapy can be as simple as hot or cold packs used at home to ease pain and swelling, or a warm, relaxing soak in the bathtub. A whirlpool bath can be used to soothe and massage the body as well as to treat circulatory problems. Saunas encourage sweating, which people believe allows the body to eliminate toxins that build up inside. Another toxin-cleansing method is drinking at least eight glasses of pure water a day.

LIGHT THERAPY

Natural light plays a vital role in regulating the biological clock of the human body. It controls sleep and hormone production. Full-spectrum light from the sun is necessary for the body's production of vitamin D, which helps with the absorption of calcium and other minerals.

Lack of light has been linked to depression, especially seasonal affective disorder, which in turn affects the quality of sleep and the immune response of the body.

Artificial light that simulates sunlight is called "bright light therapy" (BLT). To undergo BLT, a person sits directly in front of a light box every day for a period of time. The amount of time varies greatly among individuals, and it changes depending on the season of the year. Some people require as little as forty minutes a day, and they can occupy themselves with reading a book or doing another quiet activity during their therapy time.[16] Light therapy can be administered in a clinic or office environment, but home versions of full-spectrum lighting are now available at relatively low cost. Many people administer BLT to themselves at home.

AROMATHERAPY

Aromatherapy is the use of essential oils extracted from roots, flowers, leaves, and stalks of plants and absorbed into the body either through the pores of the skin during massage or by inhalation through the nose. The goal of aromatherapy is to help the body, mind, and spirit achieve balance.

The most commonly used aromatic oils include chamomile, sage, lavender, peppermint, rosemary, sandalwood, and tea tree. To find sources for aromatherapy products and other aromatherapy resources, go to the Web site of the National Association of Holistic Aromatherapy at http://www.naha.org.

LOOKING BACK

Alternative care includes many more nontoxic, noninvasive practices, theories, and disciplines than I have detailed in this chapter. It is highly important to use your discretion in choosing an alternative approach to health and wellness, since you cannot consult one trustworthy organization for certification or regulation.

At the same time, alternative care from responsible and well-trained individuals is just what the doctor ordered for complete health. Most of the methods of alternative care are designed to boost the self-healing and the immune system capacity of the human body. For the sake of your wholeness, I particularly recommend regular chiropractic adjustments from a licensed chiropractic doctor (you will see the initials "DC" after their names) for biomechanical and structural problems of the spine and joints, muscle problems, nutrition and natural health-care advice, general lack of health, and nervous system imbalances that manifest themselves with pain, numbness, tingling, or burning.

Evaluate with your doctor both what you need in terms of regular tune-ups and what is available to you in your local area. In the future, perhaps the expense of more types of alternative care will be covered by employers' insurance programs so that more people can take advantage of their resources.

☑ TO-DO LIST

☑ Schedule an appointment with a competent chiropractor in your local area.

☑ Schedule a massage with a trained massage therapist.

☑ Consider acupuncture or acupressure as an adjunct to your wellness care.

☑ Research options in your geographic area for wellness care that matches your personal needs.

☑ Make alternative care a regular part of your monthly health regimen.

Motivation: Keeping Up the Good Work

⌒

I can do all things through Christ which strengtheneth me.
—PHILIPPIANS 4:13, KJV

⌒

Without motivation, DREAM Health will be only a dream. Without motivation, the information you have learned about diet, rest, exercise, and alternative care will sit on a dusty shelf—and your health will remain as it always has been. It is one thing to learn information about how to eat right, how to get quality rest, how to get exercise, and options for alternative care; it's another thing to be consistent in applying that information to your daily decisions. But once you are motivated, you really can come into a place of the best possible health and well-being.

I believe that the startling statistics about the state of American health can be a strong source of motivation. Remember—more than 60 percent of Americans are dying of heart disease and cancer, both of which are more than 80 percent preventable through the DREAM Health lifestyle. You would never step out in front of a bus, right? You know it would do you permanent harm—or kill you. But that is what you are doing where your long-term health is concerned, if you keep stepping in front of the bus of fast food, prescription drugs, and stress-producing situations—it's a form of slow suicide.

Once you come to understand this, the motivation to change is as natural and easy as it is to avoid the bus. You see, I can't just tell you to quit smoking or eating chocolate, if you love those things. That will never work. I need to add something, not take something away from you. But if I persuade you to change your belief system, then you will choose on your own to change your behavior. You will have the motivation you need.

HOW ABOUT *YOU*?

Do you feel that you have enough energy to accomplish what you would like to do each day? Are you comfortable with your current level of health? Do you feel that you are working to your highest health potential? What will cause you to act on the information you've learned and to begin (and continue) your journey to optimum health? Let's spend some time discussing how to get motivated and how to keep your motivation high as you work toward optimum health. Remember—health is normal, and normal is optimal.

Give yourself the right message

The thoughts that you have, the people with whom you surround yourself, and the environment in which you place yourself all have an effect on your level of motivation or mental attitude. If you are constantly saying to yourself, "I can't do this," or "This is just too hard," or "I don't have time," then you will find that you cannot do what it takes to apply the principles you have learned in this book. You will complicate the process, and you won't feel that you have the time to devote to it. But if you change your internal dialogue to, "I know I can do this," or "I have the discipline to do this," or "I will find the time to do this," or even, "I am killing myself with the toxic substances I am putting into my body," then you will find that you can succeed.

You have the key to success already because it resides in your thinking processes. You can unlock success by focusing your thoughts. Your mind, when it has been educated about health-promoting principles, can link up with your natural motivation to make intelligent decisions that will enhance your overall health. Your natural motivation will help you use the components of your knowledge like a well-cared-for set of tools.

To get a better idea of how your thinking processes work, you might want to try a little experiment. All of us are constantly talking to ourselves as we carry on an internal dialogue in our thoughts. We are not aware of how much thought-processing we do. To help yourself change your limiting thoughts, keep a journal for one day. Set a timer to go off every fifteen minutes. When it rings, stop and write down whatever you were thinking. You will be amazed at all the self-defeating and unwanted thoughts you will become aware of through this exercise. Now you are better equipped to start building new habits based on your new beliefs. (The purpose of the DREAM Health program is to equip you with new beliefs that will naturally change your behavior.)

The people with whom you spend time can reinforce your self-motivation. If the human dynamics are healthy ones, the company you keep and the daily human environment in which you work and live can help you to attain and maintain optimum health. Everyone has had the experience of spending time with an individual or group of people who are uplifting, encouraging, and generally supportive of each other. Haven't you found it to be true that you come away from such an encounter feeling more light-hearted, more built up, and more positive than you were before?

Conversely, all of us have had to spend time with a very negative person or group, coming away from the experience down, even depressed, with less energy than before. The lesson is a simple one: your internal well-being is affected greatly by your external environment, especially when it involves other people. And to a large extent, you can choose where you will spend your time. Will you squander your mental, emotional, and physical health by immersing yourself in an unhealthy environment, or will you choose to spend as much time as possible in a healthier human environment?

One of the most consistent messages I convey to my two children is the importance of lifting each other up with kind and grateful hearts. I hope they never forget it as long as they live.

THE DREAM HEALTH THOUGHT PROCESS

Your mind can be extensively educated, but if you do not focus your thinking in such a way as to cooperate with the innate wisdom that your Creator has given you, your mind will not work in your favor. In fact, the same educated mind can work *against* you, depending upon how you focus your thinking. It is a matter of choice.

You can choose to focus on your hopes and dreams—in which case your fears and doubts will fade away. You can choose, if you want, to focus on your fears and doubts—in which case your hopes and dreams will fade away. You want to increase your ability to keep your focus where you want it, on your hopes and dreams.

BREAK OUT OF YOUR SELF-IMPOSED PRISON!

One of the common slogans among men and women who are serving long sentences in federal prison is "You've got nothin' comin'." It's a sad, hopeless statement, robbing the inmates of what little hope they have left....

Sadly, many people "on the outside" are living behind self-imposed bars, in prisons of their own making, and have succumbed to the same type of thinking. *This is the best you can expect. It isn't going to get any better, so you might as well sit down, keep quiet, and endure it.*

No! You can break out of that prison! The door is unlocked. All you have to do is start expecting good things in your life and start believing God for a great future. You do have good things coming![1]

—JOEL OSTEEN

Most of us are not fully aware of how our minds run amuck with all kinds of "garbage thinking." Your mind may be recycling old worries, anxieties, regrets, or emotional pain—"What if this thing happens?" "I must meet these expectations." "I'm scared to do that thing." "If only I hadn't done that." "I was hurt by that in the past." We may be reliving angry or unpleasant conversations with family members or the people we work with—"He shouldn't have said that." "She makes me so mad. I wish I had said..." We may be chastising ourselves internally—"You're so stupid. You never get it right." Or our thoughts may be preoccupied with the plot of the movie we just saw or with a report we just heard or read in the news.

Part of your success on the path to DREAM Health is to recognize how the thoughts you produce in your educated mind influence your ability to allow your innate, God-given intelligence to flow. Are you working with your God-given intelligence or against it? Earlier in the book we discussed the difference between your educated mind and your inherent mind. Your educated mind serves the very important function of enabling you to order your world, to be where you need to be, and to interact with other people.

As you start paying attention to the thoughts that you produce through your educated mind, you will then be able to make *choices* about your thoughts. Will you choose to think uplifting thoughts, or will you choose to think negative thoughts? Your optimum health reality is determined by your choices.

Of course, first you must become aware that you are so much more than the thoughts you think. Your thoughts do drive you to actions, but your spiritual connection to God is so much bigger than the self-limiting internal dialogue of your human thought processes. As you learn to put your focus on God, you can quit trying to do all the work yourself.

I like to think of an educated brain as a set of tools like the software packages on your computer. You don't use your spreadsheet software to send an e-mail, do you? And you don't use your e-mail software to create a spreadsheet. You consider the task at hand, and then you choose the appropriate application for it. In the same way, you can choose from your "brain software" the proper tools for living your life. You can become skilled at using those tools, to the point that you automatically make the healthiest choices.

Sadly, what happens to most of us is that we stay stuck in a rut—like trying to use our e-mail software to accomplish data analysis. As a consequence, it never occurs to us that we have any further capabilities. We never turn off the software that we use the most. It has become habitual to us; we never try to think or live any differently.

You need to remember that when your educated brain (the part of you that is consciously thinking, judging, categorizing, and attempting to put things in order) is in overdrive, you experience stress. As you have already learned, stress releases cortisol and adrenaline into the body, and when these hormones flood your system, they wreak havoc on all of your bodily processes, leading to adrenal failure and disease.

Your goal is to utilize the "flow" part of your brain (that portion of the brain that intrinsically knows and controls your heartbeat, nerve impulses, blood flow, breathing, and all bodily processes), which will keep your bodily processes running well. Your God-given intelligence knows everything about how your body works. You want it to be free to do its job. You want your stress-producing thought processes to stay out of the way so that your God-given intelligence can do its job effectively. You want to calm your busy mind so that you can be aware of your God-connection. This is the *ahhh* feeling of peace, that feeling you get when you let go and let God.

This approach to life may sound like a lot of work, but I can tell you from personal experience that it is worth it. It takes practice and dedication to develop an awareness of how your thoughts help or hinder you, but if you do it, you can enter into the reality that you so dearly want.

Keeping the mirror polished

Think of your brain as a mirror that reflects whatever is in front of it. What if a sunbeam (God) is shining down on your mirror? You will reflect His light, correct?

But how will that reflection look? It will be difficult for you to reflect a clear image if the mirror of your soul and mind is clouded or marred, cracked, or smudged in some way. The reflected image will be altered. You won't be able to reflect or manifest the reality of God (which is, I believe, your purpose here on Earth). Do you see how important it is to have a mirror of the highest quality?

Do you think that Jesus worked sixty hours a week, ate junk food, drank espresso and soft drinks, and handled stresses and physical problems with quick-fix drugs? Of course not! So why should we do these things?

Many people make the mistake of focusing on what they're getting in life as the problem. However, when they do that they are focusing on the mere reflection. They don't realize that what they are seeing is a reflection of something from a higher source. And they can't do much about changing a mere reflection. Even if they block part of it or refract the light further, the reflection reverts to its original state as soon as they stop trying to change it. It's as if they are treating only the symptoms of an ailment instead of finding the root problem. The root or source of the reflection is the mirror of their educated mind.

You need to pay attention to the condition of your mirror and, with God's help, polish it as much as possible. Then you will be able to truly reflect the sunbeam of His light to the world around you.

> *Let this mind be in you, which was also in Christ Jesus.*
>
> —PHILIPPIANS 2:5, KJV

You will be able to see the path in front of you, and your life will reflect an improved reality. In addition, God will be able to use you to cast a clear reflection of His love and power on your environment. Because you will no longer be cloudy or broken, you will not reflect a shadowed or fragmented light, but rather one that is sharp and clear. Your mind and soul will be healthy and filled with God's light, and your health will be self-sustaining.

Living in the now

In order to start becoming aware of what is going on in your brain, you need to be present—in the moment. Many of us live in the past, feeling guilty about what has already happened. Many others live in the future, anxious about what might happen. If you stop wandering into the past or the future and simply remain in the present, you can observe your thoughts and change them with God's help.

The past is just that—past and gone. And if you keep looking toward the future, you will never really get there, because you are always in the now. We are present-time beings. Think about it; each of us has five senses—sight, hearing, taste, touch, and smell—and all of our senses operate in the *now*. We were created to be in the *now*.

In the Bible, God speaks to Moses and instructs him to tell the Israelites, "I am that I am."

> And God said unto Moses, I AM THAT I AM: and he said, Thus shalt thou say unto the children of Israel, I AM hath sent me unto you.
>
> —Exodus 3:14, KJV

God didn't say, "I am who I was" or "I am who I will be." He said, "I am that I am." He is a God of the present moment. In God, everything is expressed in the present tense. If you want to be present with God, you need to be present in the moment, the *now*.

You will find that functioning in the present moment provides great advantages for you. If you are in the now, everything just "is." Your thoughts are not tainted by the mistakes of the past, nor are they affected by your anxieties about the future. Without so many distractions, you can better ascertain if the mirror of your soul and mind is clear enough to reflect God's light. Make it your goal to live in the "now" state.

One way to practice being in the "now" is to simply observe the world around you, without judging it. Just watch your children playing. Just look at the leaves on the trees. It is the easiest way to bring yourself into the present moment.

MOTIVATED TO DEVELOP HELPFUL HABITS

Successful attainment of your DREAM Health depends upon exercising strong willpower, or what I prefer to call "choice-power." It also depends upon developing disciplined habits. These two components are the biggies in terms of accomplishing your goal.

Willpower or choice-power

Your willpower or choice-power is your ability to control your decisions, to follow through with them. It is an energetic determination to succeed at a particular chosen task.

When you exercise your choice-power, it's as if you are flexing your spiritual muscles. And like everything else in your life, when it is coupled with God's power, your human willpower is truly amazing. No longer do you have to expend so much of your limited human energy. Martin Luther wrote, "When God works in us, the will, being changed and sweetly breathed upon by the Spirit of God, desire and acts, not from compulsion, but responsively."[2]

In essence, willpower is simply choice. That's why I like the term *choice-power*. It is not some great beast that needs to be wrestled into place—it is simply choice. When you think of it in those terms, you can relax and use it well.

Disciplined habits

You and I are creatures of habit. Our habits are unconscious patterns, and they determine what we experience and think and feel.

Did you know that as much as 90 percent of your routine behavior is based on your unconscious habits? The authors of *The Power of Focus* said, "Most of your daily activities are habits that go on day after day, year after year, often without you even being aware of them. They become firmly established as the way you do things, and they involve every area of your life including your work, family, income, health, and relationships."[3]

Our habits can be changed, because our brains are equipped with the capability of *neuroplasticity*, which means that the electrical synapses patterns can be stimulated in a new direction, thus forming new habits.

In order to make a change to a current habit, you must become aware of what your habit is, because you are largely unconscious of it. Becoming conscious of your habits takes effort, and you may need the help of your spouse or friends to see them. But becoming conscious of them is the first step toward changing them, and it is the first step toward making your own clear choices about them. You don't want to let them continue to rule your life unconsciously, unless they are habits that you have decided will be helpful.

Your goal is to form new habits, ones that you want to have. They will allow you to react reflexively—that it, by reflex, without thinking—to whatever happens around you.

It it's true that it takes about twenty-one days to change a habit, this long turnaround time results from the fact that we start out being unconscious of our habits. The first step toward changing a habit is to become aware of what your habits are. Then you decide which habits you want to address and change, which habits you may want to develop, and what barriers may be in your way. Last but not least, you can outline specific action steps that will get you to your goal of establishing a particular behavior as a good habit.

Throughout the process, you are taking responsibility for yourself—emotionally, physically, mentally, and spiritually. Responsibility means "response-ability." You have the ability to control your response to any situation. You have the ability to build new habits.

Your mind, body, and spirit are so interrelated. They are a triad, an indissolvable union, and they influence each other toward—or away from—wholeness. The better stewardship you exercise over each component, the better your connection to God will be. And the better your connection to God becomes, the more useful flow you will enjoy. If you think positive thoughts, you will enjoy better physical and mental health, and you will feel closer to God. If you entertain negative thoughts, every cell of your body will know about it. Your state of mind will have a global effect on your physical state as well as your spiritual situation. And of course, if you are compromised in your physical state or your spiritual situation, your brain will respond with increased stress and anxiety.

It's well worth it to seek to change your habits so you can reach the highest goal—wholeness in mind, body, and spirit.

BARRIERS TO CHANGE

You will find that there are some common barriers to making changes in your habits. These are so common that I want to lay them out for you, so you don't have to figure them out by the slow process of trial and error.

Grieving

A common barrier to the process of change involves grieving. Whenever you change a deeply ingrained habit (for example, cigarette smoking), you will grieve for the comfort that you gained from that habit.

You will grieve for other reasons, too. Perhaps your social life has been filled with fellow smokers. When you decide to make a change in that habit, your decision affects the other members of your group. Some of them may have a hard time with it, and they may express their disapproval to you. In addition, you will tend to lose contact with some of them because you won't share the activity of smoking any longer. Until your new, nonsmoking habit gets well established, you won't want to be in your old environment. In fact, you may never return to the places where you used to smoke. So you will miss your old friends and your familiar routines. You will grieve for the changes to your relationships, the loss of camaraderie, and likely from the lack of support from old friends. Some of your friends may decide to join you in changing the same habit. But overall, you will need to suffer some tangible losses in order to achieve a greater gain (health through not smoking). The ongoing pain of grieving your losses can make you stumble in your decision to change.

You can overcome this barrier if you allow yourself to grieve, but recognize what's going on so you don't stumble as badly. Don't get stuck in the grieving stage. Just remind yourself of your reasons for making the change in the first place, and you will find it easier to allow for the pain of the distance between you and others. You can and should look for help and support elsewhere. Seek ongoing support either with a friend who is working in the same direction, or with a specific support group geared to your goal. A support system will allow you to share progress, setbacks, experiences, and emotions.

Ultimately, we adopt habits such as smoking and overeating (which happen to be two of the largest contributing factors to the primary killer diseases in America, cancer and heart disease) to soothe ourselves, to decrease our emotional pain. Your new goal will be to enhance your connection to God, because He is the best source for the peace you crave.

Distractions

Distractions can turn out to be a big barrier to changing your habits, if you allow them to predominate. "I just can't go and work out, because the kids keep distracting me." "I have too much to do to take a fifteen-minute nap."

What if you should decide that all of your so-called distractions are merely new choices? A distraction may be something that you feel you have no control over; as a result, you tend to give it too much power. Take back the power of the distraction and stop letting it take you out of the flow of the moment—instead, view it as a new choice between focusing on the distraction and focusing on your original goal.

Your choice is a conscious one. You can let yourself be distracted and deflected from your goal of, for instance, taking a rest or getting some exercise, or you can choose to find a creative way to continue to pursue your goal. Essentially, there is no such thing as a distraction, because our so-called distractions are merely new opportunities to exercise your power of choice. With God's help, you refocus yourself and take one more step toward establishing your DREAM Health lifestyle.

Naturally, everything tends to take the path of least resistance. That's why it seems so easy to succumb to distractions. But I am here to tell you that you *can* make a conscious choice to pursue your goal. If you allow yourself to be distracted, essentially you become a victim of your circumstances; you yield to the "tyranny of the urgent." You cannot focus on what you wanted to focus on, your circumstances may plunge you into a negative frame of mind, and your pursuit of a worthy goal is deflected.

LET'S GET PRACTICAL

OK, so it is important to stay present in the moment in order to flow with God's Spirit, but how do you get there in your everyday life? Let me suggest some practical tools that may help you.

You may discover, as I did, that in the process of trying to establish new habits, your God-connection is amplified in unexpected ways. A while back, in an effort to strengthen my discipline, I started getting up at 4:30 in the morning. First, I jogged for half an hour. Next, I read a spiritual book for half an hour. Last, for another half hour I tried to visualize how I wanted my day to go. I followed this program consistently for thirty days in a row. About halfway through this process, I found that my brain was so tired that it just gave up. However, much to my delight, my inner impulses began to flow. As a result, I could more clearly perceive the difference between my educated mind and my spirit than I ever had before. I was excited to see how much more I was able to accomplish by letting my God-given intelligence do its job. Because my mind was so tired, my body automatically turned off my educated brain. Now I found that God could better guide me, because I had gotten myself out of the way. You've heard the saying, "Let go and let God." That's what happened.

Meditation

Now I meditate twice a day—once upon waking and then again right before falling asleep. I feel that it is important to meditate upon waking because it sets the tone for my brain for the rest of the day, and meditating before sleep is helpful because it clears my mind so that I can sleep more restfully. In other words, my meditation time allows me to quiet my brain and become more connected to my spirit and therefore to God's Spirit.

In the process of meditation, I think about the day to come (or the day just completed). Often I consider what plans God might have for my future, five or ten years down the road, and I ask Him to help me stay focused. I bring my concerns onto the screen of my mind and express my desire, for example, to create closer relationships with my family, to become more helpful in my professional life, or to maintain healthy habits. I pray and I thank God, most often thanking Him that my wishes and desires have already been met by His provision. My meditation is a way to keep my "mirror" clean. After I meditate in the morning, I don't have to worry about the rest of my day. I find it much more automatic to stay in the present, moment by moment.

Now I realize that many people have a negative view of meditation because of its association with Eastern occult religions, where meditation entails emptying the mind and making it a passive recipient for whatever is "out there." Some of what is out there isn't so good. But the kind of meditation I'm talking about involves filling your mind with truth based on God's Word.

And believe it or not, you already know how to meditate if you know how to put two thoughts together. Have you ever worried about something? Well, that's meditation—although I don't recommend making a habit of *that* kind of meditation!

Bill Johnson, in his book *The Supernatural Power of a Transformed Mind*, describes meditation like this:

> Every person, saint and sinner alike, meditates every day. The question is, what are you meditating on? Say you've got a problem with your finances. A person with a renewed mind derives joy even in that circumstance because joy comes not by what is seen but by what God says....
>
> But a little voice called worry steals in and reasons with you, saying, "Years ago you disobeyed the Lord financially, and now you will reap what you sowed." That might sound like a pretty good argument, and it might cause you to shift your meditation from God's Word to worry. Soon that little voice has grown so big it's like a megaphone in your ear. You forget that God said He would "keep him in perfect peace, whose mind is stayed on" Him (Isa. 26:3). Perfect peace means divine health, prosperity, wellness of being, soundness of mind. *Stayed* or *fixed* means "braced, lodged in an immovable position." But when we listen to worry, we become "unfixed." Why does worry shout so loudly for our attention? Because if we look at it long enough, it will gain our trust. Pretty soon we begin praying out of fear, and eventually we quit praying and start looking for sympathy. We have trusted that other voice, and it won the affections of our heart. [4]

The more we worry, the less in control we feel. We feel insecure; we become afraid. The more fear we experience, the more we are paralyzed. We need to establish new thought-habits, patterns of meditation, and we need to make decisions about unresolved matters, starting with the decision to trust God with them. Once we have made a decision, we don't have to worry about it anymore.

Then Jesus said to his disciples: "Therefore I tell you, do not worry about your life, what you will eat; or about your body, what you will wear. Life is more than food, and the body more than clothes. Consider the ravens: They do not sow or reap, they have no storeroom or barn; yet God feeds them. And how much more valuable you are than birds! Who of you by worrying can add a single hour to his life?"

—Luke 12:22–25

Don't forget the value of soothing music. Some people do their best praying and meditating along with specially chosen recordings of uplifting and meditative music, often instrumental (no lyrics).

Positive affirmations

Positive affirmations are statements that can help you over the hump and into new habits of thought and action. Your mind will believe what it is told, especially if the statements are repeated more than once or twice. Therefore, it is critical that we make as many positive statements to ourselves as we can and that we reinforce to ourselves the truth that we encounter during our daily reading and interactions with others.

You can create or copy actual statements and post them where you will see them. Some people type them on strips of paper. Others handwrite them on sticky notes or even tape-record them. Put the notes wherever you spend time with your mind not busy—for instance, on your bathroom mirror, in your car, on your refrigerator. We all need constant reminders, or we will forget what we're aiming for. I have a sheet of paper with many positive affirmations on it, and I say them out loud to myself twice a day.

Some people take the time to create what is called a life board. They start by going through old magazines to find pictures and words that best describe their life goals. They cut them out and glue them to paper or poster board, collage-fashion. The results can be large or small, to match personal tastes and circumstances. Some people make a large collage on poster board that they can hang on the wall; others choose to make a little card-sized collage that will fit into their pocket calendars. I have mine in my garage so that I see it every day when I drive my car in. A life board can help you focus on what is important to you, and you can add to it or subtract from it as you go through the seasons of your life.

Journaling

Equally helpful to many people as a way of sorting through their thoughts is journaling. You can find an abundance of resources about journaling in books or online.

Of course, you can keep a journal in a number of ways. You can use a simple spiral notebook or a legal pad. You can journal on your computer. Journaling is so popular these days that you can find blank journals for sale in any bookstore. Blank journals have all kinds of covers and come in all sizes, so you can look them over until you find one that you really like, one that seems to call to you to fill its pages. Keep your journal wherever you like to sit in your reflective moments. Spend a few minutes on a regular basis recording what you are thinking, what you are thankful for, and what you are hoping for. You will become more aware of your internal dialogue, and you will turn it in a positive direction.

Goal-setting

Goal-setting is a helpful tool for breaking down your major goals into more achievable steps. Effective goal-setting is an excellent method to keep yourself disciplined and motivated.

Your final goal may be to lose thirty pounds by Christmas. If you break that big goal into smaller ones that are more easily achieved, you have a much higher likelihood of success. "Achievable Goal: I will eat a balanced breakfast every day." "Achievable Goal: I will lose at least one pound this week."

After you assess the big picture and find a way to set smaller goals that you can reach on a daily or weekly basis, it will seem like no time before you will have reached your bigger goal. Daily and weekly short-term goals are more immediate, more attainable; they will help you feel successful along the way, like getting all the different belt colors or stripes on your martial arts belt on the way to becoming a black belt.

(At the end of this book, you will find DREAM Health journal pages, on which you can record your weekly health goals. The act of physically writing down your goals will help you to keep them, because the written word more easily serves as a contract with yourself. I promise you that if you can keep achieving your daily and weekly goals for three weeks, you will have succeeded, a little at a time, in changing whatever habits you set out to change.)

Before setting any goals, it is helpful to ask yourself some questions, such as "What motivates me? Is it enough to be able to check a goal I have just met off a list, or do I need to reward myself with something?" Coming to an understanding about how you tick will help you to succeed. I do believe, however, that a payoff or a win when you do hit a goal is the most effective positive reinforcement of all.

Mentors

Can you find a person or a group of people, perhaps a friend, a health-care professional, or a support group, who have already attained the goal you want to reach—or who are working on attaining the same goal? A mentor can keep you going when you think you can no longer go on. A mentor can help you realign your thinking to match your original goals. A mentor can be a generally positive influence in your life. Find someone who has what you want, and hang out with that person. Remember, you will become what you are in front of. Put yourself in front of a good mentor.

LOOKING BACK

As I said at the beginning of this chapter, without motivation, DREAM Health can only be a dream. With God's help, as you get to know yourself better and better, you can choose the right motivational tools to help you naturally and easily enter into the DREAM Health lifestyle.

Give Him permission to change you so that the mirror of your soul and mind will reflect His image to the world around you. Allow His wisdom to be your guide.

Remember that what you are in front of is what you are going to become. Keep yourself in front of God's holiness, and your life will reflect it. Keep yourself in front of the principles of wholeness, and your life will reflect it. Keep reading, keep exercising, keep maintaining a balance between work and rest, keep receiving the right messages from mentors, family, and friends, and keep on receiving good wellness-oriented care.

You are not doing this just to lose weight or to look better. You are not doing this even to be more full of energy or more muscular. You are doing it for a lifestyle. You are choosing a different path from the world around you, which wants you to look like a professional model even though it also tells you to supersize your fast food. You are turning a blind eye to advertisements and the frantic pace around you. You, like Jesus, are in the world but not part of the world (John 17:14).

Attaining and maintaining optimum health will take time, commitment, and perseverance, but it's worth every effort. After a while, you may reach a sort of plateau in your ability to change. Don't lose sight of your goal, which is to achieve a supernaturally natural lifestyle of wholeness.

☑ TO-DO LIST

☑ Make time each day to journal about your habits and your choices.

☑ Record your personal goals in your journal.

☑ Read the Bible or an inspirational book.

☑ Take some quiet time in the morning and in the evening to meditate.

☑ Each day, write down two negative thoughts and find a way to make them positive.

☑ Get a timer, and try the internal dialogue exercise.

Nutrition Helps

In this appendix you will find information to help you achieve DREAM Health.

DREAM HEALTH NATURAL FOOD PYRAMID

REFINED SUGAR*
0%

WHOLE GRAINS
5%

SUPPLEMENTS
Liquid multivitamin and omega-3, -6, and -9 fatty acids

NUTS AND LEGUMES
15%

LEAN ORGANIC MEATS
(chicken and beef)
20%

ORGANIC FRUITS AND VEGETABLES
60%

WATER
Divide body weight by two and drink that
amount in ounces daily

---

* Refined sugars are never recommended and minimally tolerated.

Foods to Avoid[1]

- Fried foods (fries, doughnuts, chips, etc.)
- Products made from processed flour (white breads, pasta, etc.)
- Caffeinated beverages
- All nonorganic produce, including dried fruits
- Dairy products (limited non-pasteurized OK)
- Sweet juices
- Tap water
- Alcoholic beverages
- Sprayed, early-harvested fruits and vegetables
- Grain-fed, hormone- or antibiotic-laced meats
- Smoked meats
- Pork (high fat; can carry parasites, mold spores)
- Farm-raised fish (higher toxicity, lower omega-3)
- Tuna (top of the food chain; accumulates mercury from other fish)
- Shellfish (bottom-feeders, accumulate toxins)
- Soy products (limited, if fermented)
- Hydrogenated and partially hydrogenated fats
- Added salt
- MSG or hydrolyzed protein (disguised MSG)
- White sugar
- Aspartame and other artificial sweeteners
- All chemical food additives and colors
- High fructose corn syrup
- Non-fiber carbohydrate additives (sugar, fructose)

MAIL-ORDER SUPPLIERS OF MEATS[2]

An online search can provide you with additional sources for free-range and wild meats.

Free-range meats

- Bering Pacific Ranch (Alaska)—www.naturesfirst.net/productinfo.html
- Coleman Natural Beef (Colorado)—www.colemannatural.com
- Dakota Natural Beef (North Dakota)—www.dakotabeefcompany.com
- Laura's Lean Beef—www.laurasleanbeef.com
- North Hollow Farms (Vermont)—www.naturalmeat.com
- Rains Natural Meats (Missouri)—www.rainsnaturalmeats.com
- Van Wie Natural Foods (New York)—www.vanwienaturalmeats.com

Game meat

- Game Sales International (Colorado)—www.gamesalesintl.com
- Gem Farms Buffalo (New York)—www.gemfarmsbuffalo.com
- MacFarlane Farms (Wisconsin)—www.pheasant.com
- Mount Royal Game Meat (Texas)—www.mountroyal.com
- Mountain America Jerky (Colorado)—www.mountainamericajerky.com
- New West Foods (Colorado)—www.newwestfoods.com
- Seattle's Finest Exotic Meats (Washington)—www.exoticmeats.com

NATURAL REMEDIES GUIDE[1]

Disease/ Affliction	Medical Approach	Natural Alternatives
Acid reflux; gas; heartburn	Prilosec	Reduce stress; reduce dietary fats/ sugars; adopt vegetable diet; add probiotics; chiropractic adjustment of sixth thoracic vertebra; slippery elm
Allergies	Claritin; Allegra	Liver cleanser; amylase; chiropractic adjustment of second and first cervical vertebra
Angina	Nitroglycerin	L-carnitine; coenzyme Q_{10}; magnesium; hawthorn; khella
Anxiety; stress	Prozac	Liquid multivitamin with B-complex; exercise; relaxation techniques; meditation; regular rest/naps; balance life schedule; sunshine; liquid multivitamin; MSM
Arthritis	Celebrex	Massage; chiropractic adjustments; deep-stretching routines; yoga; no-sugar liquid multivitamin; MSM
Asthma	Theophylline; corticosteriods	Adjust third thoracic vertebra; relieve stress; build immune system (also see Allergies)

NATURAL REMEDIES GUIDE[1]		
Disease/ Affliction	**Medical Approach**	**Natural Alternatives**
Autism; ADD	Ritalin	Multivitamin supplementation; vitamin B_6; omega-3 oil; chiropractic adjustments
Back pain	Celebrex; muscle relaxers; acetaminophen; tricyclic antidepressants	Chiropractic adjustments; massage; exercise; yoga; core strength and stress-reduction techniques; MSM
Benign prostatic hypertrophy	Alpha blockers	Saw palmetto
Bladder infection	Antibiotics	Cranberry juice; vitamin C; raw apple cider vinegar; watermelon juice
Carpal tunnel syndrome	Anti-inflammatories; corticosteriods	Massage; chiropractic adjustments; vitamin B_6; stretch hands toward back of elbows

NATURAL REMEDIES GUIDE[1]		
Disease/ Affliction	*Medical Approach*	*Natural Alternatives*
Cancer	Chemo-therapy; radiation	Strengthen immune system with folic acid; vitamin D; flaxseed; grapes; sulphane; turmeric; rosemary; licorice; ginseng; bromelain; ellagic acid; citrus juice; papaw tree bark; blue/green algae; probiotics; OPC calcium; proper diet; rest; exercise; alternative care; DREAM Health lifestyle
Chronic fatigue syndrome	Anti-inflam-matories; antihista-mines; anti-depressants; codeine	Massage therapy; chiropractic adjustment; exercise; rest; mental/ spiritual stimulation; building immune system; ginseng + multivitamins; DREAM Health lifestyle
Circulation problems	Pentoxi-fylline	Vitamin E; omega-3 fatty acids; liquid multivitamin; cardiovascular exercise
Cold sores; herpes viruses	Valtrex; Abreva	Deglycyrrhizinated licorice; acidophilus; calendula; vitamins B_1 and B_2; lysine
Colds	Nasal decon-gestants; Sudafed	Strengthen immune system with vitamin C; rest; green tea; chiropractic adjustment; echinacea; zinc; ginseng
Consti-pation	Laxatives	Drink 1 oz. of water for every pound of body weight; eat prunes; GastroZyme + acidophilus; psyllium husks; probiotics
Diabetes (type 2)	Insulin	Chromium; ginseng; garlic; onion; bitter melon; bilberry; vitamin E; biotin; lypoic acid; whole-food diet of vegetables/ fruits; exercise; reduce stress; DREAM Health lifestyle

NATURAL REMEDIES GUIDE[1]		
Disease/ Affliction	*Medical Approach*	*Natural Alternatives*
Ear infection	Acetaminophen	Chiropractic adjustment to first and second cervical vertebrae; natural glycerin oil drops; mullen oil; garlic oil
Fibromyalgia	Muscle relaxers; painkillers	Chiropractic adjustments; massage therapy; yoga; stretching; DREAM Health lifestyle
Gallbladder problems	Ursodiol; chenodiol	Reduce intake of fat, sugar, and soft drinks; colon cleanser; liver cleanser; GastroZyme; dandelion; milk thistle and acidophilus
Gout	Colchicine; corticosteriods; ACTH	Folic acid; fish oil; vitamins E and A; selenium; bromelain; cherry juice; celery juice
Heart disease	Beta blockers; ACE inhibitors	Cardiovascular exercise; reduce intake of animal fats; eat raw organic fruits and vegetables; omega-3 fatty acids; liquid multivitamin; DREAM Health lifestyle
High blood pressure	Diuretics	Garlic; coenzyme Q_{10}; fish oil; calcium; magnesium; potassium; vitamin C
High cholesterol	Calcium channel blockers; statins	Garlic; red yeast rice; niacin (vitamin B_3); fiber soy protein + cinnamon
Impotence	Viagra; Cialis	L-carnitine; liquid multivitamin with B-complex

NATURAL REMEDIES GUIDE[1]		
Disease/ Affliction	*Medical Approach*	*Natural Alternatives*
Inflammation; pain	Anti-inflammatories; painkillers	Increase water intake (divide your body weight by two and drink that amount in ounces every day); reduce nitrate intake; glucosamine; chondroitin; MSM; chiropractic adjustments; massage therapy; yoga
Insomnia	Lunesta	Valerian and melatonin
Irritable bowel syndrome	Atreza oral	Peppermint oil; GastroZyme; acidophilus + colon cleanser; no sugar
Leg pain	Cryoplasty; aspirin	Massage therapy; chiropractic adjustments; vitamins B_6 and B_{12}; electrolytes; stretching
Menopausal symptoms	Hormone replacement therapy	Black cohosh; soy protein; isoflavonoids; vitamins E and C; omega-3 oil; bioflavonoids; balanced diet; rest; exercise; multivitamins
Menstrual pain	Progestin; anti-inflammatories	Black cohosh; soy protein; isoflavonoids; vitamins E and C; omega-3 oil; bioflavonoids; balanced diet; rest; exercise; multivitamins

NATURAL REMEDIES GUIDE[1]		
Disease/ Affliction	*Medical Approach*	*Natural Alternatives*
Mid-back pain	Anti-inflammatories; painkillers	Chiropractic adjustments; massage therapy; stretching; ice (if acute); heat (if chronic); posture correction
Migraine headache	Imitrex	Chiropractic care; massage therapy; relaxation techniques; ice; no dairy
Nausea	Dramamine	Ginger; vitamin B_6
Neck pain	Acetaminophen; anti-inflammatories	Chiropractic adjustments; massage; stretching; ice (if acute); heat (if chronic); posture correction
Night vision impairment	LASIK surgery	Bilberry; leutin
Obesity	Xenical; Meridia	Cardiovascular exercise; colon cleanser and colon hydrotherapy + GastroZyme; whole raw foods; no refined sugar; carrot juice; fasting

NATURAL REMEDIES GUIDE[1]		
Disease/ Affliction	*Medical Approach*	*Natural Alternatives*
Osteoarthritis	Celebrex; Motrin	Glucosamine; chondroitin; MSM; niacin; yoga; stretching; chiropractic care; deep tissue massage therapy
Osteoporosis	Boniva; Evista	Calcium; vitamin D; ipriflavone; trace minerals; fish oil; GLA
Plantar Fasciitis	Anti-inflammatories; cortisone	Ice; stretching calf; rolling foot on golf ball; podiatric orthotics
PMS	Ibuprofen; painkillers	Chiropractic adjustments to the third lumbar vertebra; massage therapy; calcium; chaste berry; vitamin E; magnesium; multivitamin and mineral supplements; gingko
Ringing in ears	Campral; hydrocortisone drops	Vinpocetine; chiropractic adjustment; decrease inflammation
Psoriasis	Salicylic acid	Fish oil; aloe vera cream; chromium; selenium; vitamin E; burdock; red clover; milk thistle; low (2 percent) solution of Compound W; colon cleanser

NATURAL REMEDIES GUIDE[1]		
Disease/ Affliction	*Medical Approach*	*Natural Alternatives*
Shoulder pain	Anti-inflammatories; painkillers	Stretching; rehabilitative exercises; ice (if acute); heat (if chronic)
Sore throat	Ibuprofen	Increase vitamin C; natural cough drops; gargle with salt water
Stress headache	Antidepressants; beta-blockers	Chiropractic adjustment to upper cervical area; stretching; massage; ice; relaxation techniques
Ulcers	Tagamet; Prilosec	Aloe vera juice; multivitamin; chiropractic adjustment to sixth thoracic vertebra; GastoZyme; acidophilus
Varicose veins	Polidocanol	Horse chestnut; OPC; bilberry

D·R·E·A·M

My DREAM Health Journal

My DREAM Health Journal

GOALS—WEEK ONE

The goal from each of the five DREAM Health elements that I will incorporate into my life this week is:

Diet

_____

_____

_____

Rest

_____

_____

_____

Exercise

_____

_____

_____

Alternative care

_____

_____

_____

Motivation

_____

_____

_____

Steps I will take to make each goal a success

_____

_____

_____

REFLECTIONS—WEEK ONE

Use this space to record your thoughts and observations about how the goals you have set for this week are working for you. Record any positive information that you have received this week. Note any obstacles that you may have encountered in keeping your goals.

_____

_____

_____

_____

_____

_____

_____

_____

_____

_____

_____

_____

My DREAM Health Journal

The goal from each of the five DREAM Health elements that I will incorporate into my life this week is:

Diet

_____

_____

_____

Rest

_____

_____

_____

Exercise

_____

_____

_____

Alternative care

_____

_____

_____

Motivation

_____

_____

_____

Steps I will take to make each goal a success

_____

_____

_____

REFLECTIONS—WEEK TWO

Use this space to record your thoughts and observations about how the goals you have set for this week are working for you. Record any positive information that you have received this week. Note any obstacles that you may have encountered in keeping your goals.

_____

_____

_____

_____

_____

_____

_____

_____

_____

_____

_____

_____

_____

_____

_____

My DREAM Health Journal

GOALS—WEEK THREE

The goal from each of the five DREAM Health elements that I will incorporate into my life this week is:

Diet

_____

_____

_____

Rest

_____

_____

_____

Exercise

_____

_____

_____

Alternative care

_____

_____

_____

Motivation

_____

_____

_____

Steps I will take to make each goal a success

_____

_____

_____

REFLECTIONS—WEEK THREE

Use this space to record your thoughts and observations about how the goals you have set for this week are working for you. Record any positive information that you have received this week. Note any obstacles that you may have encountered in keeping your goals.

_____

_____

_____

_____

_____

_____

_____

_____

_____

_____

_____

_____

_____

_____

_____

My DREAM Health Journal

GOALS—WEEK FOUR

The goal from each of the five DREAM Health elements that I will incorporate into my life this week is:

Diet

_____

_____

_____

Rest

_____

_____

_____

Exercise

_____

_____

_____

Alternative care

_____

_____

_____

Motivation

_____

_____

_____

Steps I will take to make each goal a success

_____

_____

_____

REFLECTIONS—WEEK FOUR

Use this space to record your thoughts and observations about how the goals you have set for this week are working for you. Record any positive information that you have received this week. Note any obstacles that you may have encountered in keeping your goals.

_____

_____

_____

_____

_____

_____

_____

_____

_____

_____

_____

_____

_____

_____

_____

My DREAM Health Journal

GOALS—WEEK FIVE

The goal from each of the five DREAM Health elements that I will incorporate into my life this week is:

Diet

_____

_____

_____

Rest

_____

_____

_____

Exercise

_____

_____

_____

Alternative care

_____

_____

_____

Motivation

_____

_____

_____

Steps I will take to make each goal a success

_____

_____

_____

REFLECTIONS—WEEK FIVE

Use this space to record your thoughts and observations about how the goals you have set for this week are working for you. Record any positive information that you have received this week. Note any obstacles that you may have encountered in keeping your goals.

_____

_____

_____

_____

_____

_____

_____

_____

_____

_____

_____

_____

_____

CHAPTER 1—DREAM HEALTH: A WAY OF LIFE

1. Modified from James L. Chestnut, BEd, MSc, DC, *The Innate Diet and Natural Hygiene* (Victoria, BC, Canada: The Wellness Practice, 2004), 14.

2. Ibid.

3. Medicine.net, http://www.medterms.com/script/main/art .asp?articlekey=33613 (accessed 5/23/06).

4. Study results reviewed on August 9, 2004 by HealthGrades, a health-care quality company, for the years 2000, 2001, and 2002. See "In-Hospital Deaths from Medical Errors at 195,000 per Year USA" in *Medical News Today*, http://www.medicalnewstoday.com/ medicalnews.php?newsid=11856 (accessed 5/23/06). Original study by Drs. Chunliu Zhan and Marlene R. Miller published in the *Journal of the American Medical Association* in October of 2003. The complete study can be found at http://www.heathgrades.com.

5. Ibid.

6. As quoted on the Danish health Web site MayDay, http:// www.mayday-info.dk (accessed 5/11/06) and on related health-care -monitoring Web sites.

7. Paul Zane Pilzer, *The Wellness Revolution* (New York: John Wiley & Sons, 2002), 2.

8. Ibid.

9. Modified from Chestnut, *The Innate Diet and Natural Hygiene*, 18.

CHAPTER 2—UNPLUGGING FROM THE MATRIX

1. National Center for Health Statistics (NCHS), National Vital Statistics System (Centers for Disease Control and Prevention), "10 Leading Causes of Death, United States: All Races, Both Sexes," http://webapp.cdc.gov (accessed 4/25/06).

2. Gary Null, et al., "Death by Medicine," October 2003 http://garynull.com/Documents/deathbymedicine1.html (accessed 4/25/06).

3. Quoted from synopsis of Andrea Knox, "System to Control Deadly Drug Interaction Failing," *The Star* (Ventura County), January 7, 2001, http://www.cancure.org/medical_errors.htm (accessed 4/25/06).

4. Liz Szabo, "Insomnia Drugs: A Wake-Up Call?" *USA Today*, April 23, 2006, http://www.usatoday.com/news/health/2006-04-23 -insomnia-drugs_x.htm (accessed 4/26/06).

5. Katharine Greider, *The Big Fix: How the Pharmaceutical Industry Rips Off American Consumers* (New York: PublicAffairs/ Perseus, 2003), as quoted in "Think Prescription Drugs Are Safer and More Scientifically Proven Than Supplements? Think Again," an article by Brian W. Vaszily at Mercola.com, http://www .mercola.com/2003/aug/2/prescription_drugs.htm (accessed 4/28/06).

6. Ibid.

7. National Institutes of Health, http://www.nlm.nih.gov/ medlineplus/druginfo/medmaster/a685001.html (accessed 5/4/06).

8. "Antibacterial Drug Losing Effectiveness," February 19, 2003, as abstracted on Associated Press Archive Web site, http:// n.newsbank.com/nl-search/we/Archives (accessed 4/29/06).

9. World Health Organization, http://www.who.int/research/ en/ (accessed 5/4/06).

10. David Heymann, "Treat Now—While We Have the Drugs,"

World Health Organization Bulletin 80, no. 3 (2002), 253, cited 26 April 2006, http://www.scielosp.org/scielo.php?script=sci_ arttext&pid=S0042-96862002000300014&lng=en&nrm=iso (accessed 4/29/06).

11. From summary of chapter 8, "Rational Use of Medicines," in WHO publication *World Medicines Situation, 2004*. Archived at http://hinfo198.tempdomainname.com/medicinedocs/library .fcgi?e=d-0edmweb—00-1-0—010—4—0—0-10l—1en-5000—50 -about-0—01131-00115ERnz+VC9ee84d6400000000436f372a- 0utfZz-8-0-0&a=d&c=edmweb&cl=CL2.1.6&d=Js6160e.10 (accessed 4/29/06).

12. Ibid.

13. Greg Critser, *Generation Rx: How Prescription Drugs Are Altering American Minds, Lives, and Bodies* (New York: Houghton Mifflin, 2005).

14. Pilzer, *The Wellness Revolution*, 21.

15. Ray Moynihan, "Who Pays for the Pizza?" *British Medical Journal*, May 2003, quoted in "Health Care Update," *Today's Chiropractic*, November/December 2003, http://www .todayschiropractic.com/archives/nov_dec_03/nd2003_healthcare .html (accessed 4/26/06).

16. Ibid.

CHAPTER 3—HOW TO HANDLE STRESS

1. "The Epidemic of the Eighties," *TIME* magazine cover, June 6, 1983, the American Institute of Stress, http://www.stress.org/ problem.htm (accessed 5/4/06).

2. Information from the Medline Plus Medical Encyclopedia, a service of the U.S. National Library of Medicine and the National Institutes of Health, http://www.nlm.nih.gov/medlineplus/ency/ article/001942.htm (accessed 5/6/06).

3. Scott Hannen, DC, *Healing by Design: Unlocking Your Body's Potential to Heal Itself* (Lake Mary, FL: Siloam, 2003), 110–11.

4. The terms *allostasis* and *allostatic load* have been popularized and explored by Dr. Bruce S. McEwen, neuroendocrinology professor at Rockefeller University, New York, who is a pioneer in the field of stress research.

5. As expressed by William B. Salt II on the MindBodySpirit Medicine Web site (Parkview Publishing, Columbus, OH), http://72.14.207.104/search?q=cache:pkq8oENiNAEJ:www. parkviewpub.com/stress_response.cfm+allostasis&hl=en&gl= us&ct=clnk&cd=9 (accessed 5/5/06).

6. Steven Sauter, et al., "Stress at Work," The National Institute for Occupational Safety and Health, http://www.cdc.gov/niosh/ stresswk.html (accessed 5/4/06).

7. Ibid.

8. Ibid.

9. T. Pretrus and B. H. Kleiner, "New Developments Concerning Workplace Safety Training: Managing Stress Arising From Work," *Management Research News*, June 2003, 68–76, abstracted at IngentaConnect, http://www.ingentaconnect.com/content/mcb/02 1/2003/00000026/00000006/art00005;jsessuinis=67mt15661pua7 .alice (accessed 5/6/06).

10. John Newman, *How to Stay Cool, Calm and Collected When the Pressure's On* (New York: American Management Association, 1992), 30–31.

11. Audrey Pihulyk, "Stress, Obstacle or Opportunity," digital article published on June 22, 2001 by the Possibilities Network, http://www.possibilitiesnetwork.com/articles_links/stress.pdf (accessed 5/6/06).

12. From online article, "Good Stress, Bad Stress," *Management Issues News*, July 7, 2004, http://www.management-issues.com/ display_page.asp?section=research&id=1389 (accessed 5/4/06).

13. Drs. Redford and Virginia Williams, *In Control* (Emmaus, PA: Rodale, 2006), as quoted in Heather Cabot (ABC News), "Keys to Managing On-the-Job Stress," http://abcnews.go.com/Health/story?id=1487215 (accessed 5/8/06).

14. Ibid.

15. Cabot, "Keys to Managing On-the-Job Stress."

CHAPTER 4—DIET: KEYS TO A BALANCED APPROACH

1. Statistics from the National Health and Nutrition Examination Survey for 1999–2002, as reported by the Centers for Disease Control and Prevention, http://www.cdc.gov/nccdphp/dnpa/obesity/faq.htm#adults (accessed 5/25/06).

2. Results for a McDonald's Quarter Pounder with Cheese, with a large fries, calculated at FastFoodCalories.com, the Fast Food Nutrition Fact Explorer, at http://www.fatcalories.com/results (accessed 5/25/06).

3. Learn about probiotics on the informative Web site USProbiotics.org.

4. "Dietary Reference Intakes: Water, Potassium, Sodium, Chloride, and Sulfate" (Press Release), Institute of Medicine, February 11, 2004, http://www.iom.edu/CMS/3788/3969/18495.aspx (accessed 5/26/06).

5. "Report Sets Dietary Intake Levels for Water, Salt, and Potassium to Maintain Health and Reduce Chronic Disease Risk" (Press Release), Institute of Medicine, February 11, 2004, http://www4.nationalacademies.org/news.nsf/isbn/0309091691?OpenDocument (accessed 5/26/06).

6. "What About Grass-Fed Beef?" The Food Revolution, http://www.foodrevolution.org/grassfedbeef.htm (accessed 5/25/06).

7. Hannen, *Healing by Design*, 195.

8. Chestnut, *The Innate Diet and Natural Hygiene*, 130–155.

9. Dan Putnam, Michael Russelle, Steve Orloff, et al. (Brochure), "Alfalfa, Wildlife, and the Environment: The Importance and Benefits of Alfalfa in the 21st Century," (Novato, CA: California Alfalfa and Forage Association, 2001), 4, http://alfalfa.ucdavis.edu/subpages/Wildlife/BrochureFINAL.pdf (accessed 5/29/06).

10. Agricultural Research Service, U.S. Department of Agriculture, Food and Nutrition Research Briefs (January 2004), reporting on results of a two-nation study published in *Diabetes Care* 26, (December, 2003), 3215–3218, http://www.ars.usda.gov/is/np/fnrb/fnrb0104.htm#pinch (accessed 5/30/06).

11. William Gavin, *No White at Night: The Three Rule Diet* (New York: Riverhead, 2004).

CHAPTER 5—REST: VITAL TO YOUR HEALTH

1. Hannen, *Healing by Design*, 111.

2. Jorge Cruise, *8 Minutes in the Morning* (Emmaus, PA: Rodale, 2000), 46.

3. Amanda Gardner, *HealthScoutNews*, Norwalk, Connecticut, January 1, 2003.

4. As reported at "Wake Up to the Risks of Drowsy Driving," posted by Consumers Union of U.S., Inc. at http://www.consumerreports.org (accessed 7/19/06).

5. National Sleep Foundation (NSF), 2005 Sleep in America poll, report filed at http://www.sleepfoundation.org/_content/hottopics/2005_summary_of_findings.pdf (accessed 5/1/06).

6. National Sleep Foundation (NSF), 2006 Sleep in America poll, report filed at http://www.sleepfoundation.org/_content/hottopics/2006_summary_of_findings.pdf (accessed 5/1/06).

7. As reported at "Driving While Drowsy…Are You at Risk?" a report posted by the George Mason University Center for Advancement of Public Health in Fairfax, Virginia, http://www

.safety.gmu.edu/TS2004/pdf/yawn.pdf (accessed 5/1/06).

8. From National Highway Traffic Safety Administration, "Drowsy Driving and Automobile Crashes," Findings Report of the Gallup Organization's National Survey of Distracted and Drowsy Driving Attitudes and Behaviors, vol. 1 (2002), http://www.nhtsa .dot.gov/people/injury/drowsy_driving1/survey-distractive03/ (accessed 5/1/06).

9. As cited in "Driving While Drowsy…Are You at Risk?"

10. NIH News (National Institutes of Health), March 25, 2004, News Release filed at http://www.nhlbi.nih.gov/new/press/04-03-25.htm (accessed 5/1/06).

11. Najib T. Ayas, et al., "A Prospective Study of Sleep Duration and Coronary Heart Disease in Women," *Archives of Internal Medicine* 163(2) (2003): 205–209, as cited in Jeanie Lerche Davis, "Sleep, Less and More, Linked to Heart Disease: Too Much or Too Little Sleep Can Raise Blood Pressure, Stress Hormones," WebMD Medical News, http://www.webmd.com/content/Article/59/66895 .htm (accessed 5/3/06).

12. Gerald Rosen, presentation under the auspices of the American Academy of Sleep Medicine, http://www.aasmnet.org/ MEDSleep/Products/(RosenG)Deprivation.ppt (accessed 5/4/06).

13. Ibid.

14. Information found on Helpguide: Active Healthy Lifestyles, "Getting the Sleep You Need: Sleep Stages, Sleep Tips, and Aids," http://www.helpguide.org/life/sleeping.htm (accessed 5/1/06).

15. Ibid.

16. Burle Pettibone, DC, Chiropractic Association Conference, Tacoma, WA, March 3, 2003.

17. *Psychiatry and Clinical Neurosciences* 52 (1998): 327–332.

18. *New England Journal of Medicine* 332 (1995): 767–773.

19. From the online book *The Dark Side of Sleeping Pills* by Daniel Kripke, as cited in "Sleep Deprivation: The Great American

Myth," by Robin Lloyd, Fox News/Science, March 23, 2006, http://www.foxnews.com/story/0,2933,188924,00.html (accessed 5/1/06).

20. Ibid.

21. National Sleep Foundation 2005 Sleep in America poll.

22. Ann Hatchitt, "Taking a Vacation Benefits Employees, Employers," *Austin Business Journal*, online edition, http://www.bizjournals.com/austin/stories/2002/08/12/focus2.html (accessed 5/3/06).

23. As quoted on the Web site of Christian Aid, an interfaith organization in the United Kingdom and Ireland, http://www.christianaid.co.uk/worship/512tsu/prayer.htm (accessed 5/2/06).

24. Robert A. Schuller, *Possibility Living: Add Years to Your Life and Life to Your Years with God's Health Plan* (New York: HarperCollins/HarperSanFrancisco, 2000), 105–106.

CHAPTER 6—EXERCISE: KEEPING STRONG AND HEALTHY

1. Frank W. Booth, et al., "Waging War on Physical Inactivity Using Modern Molecular Ammunition Against an Ancient Enemy," *Journal of Applied Physiology* 93 (July 2002): 3–30.

2. Facts collected from publications of the U.S. Department of Health and Human Services (HHS); Centers for Disease Control and Prevention (CDC); Healthy People 2010 (HP2010); the National Center for Health Statistics; and Reports of the Surgeon General of the United States (SG) and published by The President's Council on Physical Fitness and Sports, http://www.fitness.gov/hbpa.htm (accessed 5/31/06).

3. JoAnn E. Mason, et al., "The Escalating Pandemics of Obesity and Sedentary Lifestyle: A Call to Action for Clinicians," *Archives of Internal Medicine* 164(3) (February 9, 2004): 249–258, abstracted at http://archinte.ama-assn.org/cgi/content/abstract/164/3/249 (accessed 6/5/06).

4. Harvard Center for Cancer Prevention, "Volume III: Prevention of Colon Cancer in the US," *Cancer Causes and Control* 10(3) (June 1999): 167–180, http://www.hsph.harvard.edu/cancer/ cancers/colon/resources/crc_insuranceguide/CRC_Guide_ Rational.pdf (accessed 6/5/06).

5. Quoted from a 2002 lecture sponsored by the National Cancer Institute, in the article "Exercise Is Key to Breast Cancer Prevention," by Peggy Vaughn, *NIH Record*, National Institutes of Health, September 17, 2002, http://www.nih.gov/news/ NIH-Record/09_17_2002/story02.htm (accessed 5/31/06).

6. Ibid.

7. As reported in the journal *Pediatrics* and in the *Healthday* article "Fit Teens May Be Safer Teens," by Robert Preidt, April 4, 2006, http://www.nlm.nih.gov/medlineplus/news/fullstory_31896. html (accessed 5/31/06).

8. Major Leo Mahony, MPT, "The Mind-Body Connection," *Hooah Magazine* online, http://www.hooah4health.com/mind/ stressmgmt/stressexercise.htm (accessed 5/31/06).

9. E. B. Larson, et al., "Exercise Is Associated with Reduced Risk for Incident Dementia Among Persons 65 Years of Age and Older," *Annals of Internal Medicine* 144 (2006), 73–81, as summarized in "Physical Fitness Can Fight Off Dementia," by Dr. Robert W. Griffith, *Health and Age*, February 13, 2006, http://www .healthandage.com (accessed 5/31/06).

10. Ibid.

11. Mahoney, "The Mind-Body Connection."

12. Ibid.

13. As reported in *Annals of Behavioral Medicine* 21(3) (1999), and in the press release, "Exercise Protects Against Symptoms of Stress," Center for the Advancement of Health, November 9, 1999, http://www.bhns.org/newsrelease/exercise11-9-99.cfm (accessed 5/31/06).

14. Lynette L. Craft, et al., "The Benefits of Exercise for the Clinically Depressed," *The Primary Care Companion to the Journal of Clinical Psychiatry* 6(3) (2004): 104–111, from abstract at http://www.pubmedcentral.gov/articlerender.fcgi?artid=474733 (accessed 5/31/06). Emphasis added.

15. Ethel S. Siris, et al., "Indication and Fracture Outcomes of Undiagnosed Low Bone Mineral Density in Post-Menopausal Women: Results from the National Osteoporosis Risk Assessment," *Journal of the American Medical Association* 286 (December 12, 2001): 2815–2822, http://jama.ama-assn.org/content/vol286/issue22/index.dtl (accessed 6/5/06).

16. Hannen, *Healing by Design*, 150.

17. "Physical Activity and Health: A Report of the Surgeon General," National Center for Chronic Disease Prevention and Health Promotion, November 17, 1999, summary at http://www.cdc.gov/nccdphp/sgr/summ.htm (accessed 5/31/06).

18. William D. McArdle, Frank I. Katch, and Victor L. Katch, *Exercise Physiology: Energy, Nutrition, and Human Performance* (Philadelphia: Lippincott Williams & Wilkins, 2004).

19. Some experts advise that you stretch before warming up; others insist you should warm up first. Whichever order you choose, you should give a few stretches to all parts of your body. Stretch alternate calf muscles first with your knee bent and then with it straight. Stretch your hamstrings (back of your thigh) by propping each leg on a nearly waist-high surface and leaning forward. Stretch your quadriceps (front of thigh) by standing up straight and catching hold of each ankle in turn, pulling your foot up behind your buttock. You may need to hang onto something for balance. Stretch your hips by "lunging" forward on alternate legs, or, if you can lie down in your exercise location, you can lie on your back with your knees bent and assume a "frog" position. You can also hold your bent knees together and rotate your lower trunk so

that your lower knee touches the ground, while keeping your upper body lying flat. Illustrations of stretching exercises are readily available in books, pamphlets, and online. (See, for example, http://www.med.umich.edu/1libr/sma/sma_stretch_art.htm.)

CHAPTER 7—ALTERNATIVE CARE: YOUR BEST HEALTH INSURANCE

1. Medline Plus, National Library of Medicine, s.v. "alternative medicine," http://www.nlm.nih.gov/medlineplus/mplusdictionary .html (accessed 6/7/06).

2. Hannen, *Healing by Design*, 136, based on James Strong, ed., *The New Strong's Exhaustive Concordance of the Bible* (Nashville: Thomas Nelson, 1997), s.v. *"pharmakeia."*

3. John A. Astin, "Why Patients Use Alternative Medicine: Results of a National Study," *Journal of the American Medical Association* 279(19) (May 20, 1998): 1548–1553, as reported in *Stanford Online Report*, May 1998, http://news-service.stanford .edu/news/1998/may27/altmedsurvey.html (accessed 6/6/06).

4. Ibid.

5. D. M. Eisenberg, et al., "Unconventional Medicine in the United States: Prevalence, Costs and Patterns of Use," *New England Journal of Medicine* 328(4) (January 28, 1993): 246–252, and D. M. Eisenberg, et al., "Trends in Alternative Medicine Use in the United States, 1990–1997: Results of a Follow-up National Survey," *Journal of the American Medical Association* 280(18) (November 11, 1998): 1551–1640, as cited in "Alternative Medicine: The Mainstreaming of the Holistic Health Movement," by Paul C. Reisser, Statement DN-395 of the Christian Research Institute, Charlotte, NC, http://www.equip.org/free/DN395.htm (accessed 6/12/06).

6. Wayne B. Jonas, "Alternative Medicine—Learning From the Past, Examining the Present, Advancing to the Future," *Journal of the American Medical Association* 280(18) (November 11, 1998):

1616–1618, as quoted in David L. Phillips, "The Dramatic Rise in the Use of Alternative Medicine," Suite101.com, March 6, 2001, http://www.suite101.com/article.cfm/chiropractic_health_care/57193 (accessed 6/7/06).

7. From the National Center for Complementary and Alternative Medicine (NCCAM), "Manipulative and Body-Based Practices: An Overview," http://nccam.nih.gov/health/backgrounds/manipulative.htm (accessed 6/12/06), citing the following studies: Astin, "Why Patients Use Alternative Medicine: Results of a National Study"; Eisenberg, et al., "Unconventional Medicine in the United States: Prevalence, Costs and Patterns of Use"; B. G. Druss and R. A. Rosenheck, "Association Between Use of Unconventional Therapies and Conventional Medical Services," *Journal of the American Medical Association* 282(7) (1999): 651–656; H. Ni, et al., "Utilization of Complementary and Alternative Medicine by United States Adults: Results from the 1999 National Health Interview Survey," *Medical Care* 40(4) (2002): 353–358; P. Barnes, et al., "Complementary and Alternative Medicine Use Among Adults: United States 2002," CDC Advance Data Report #343 (2004).

8. "Basic Techniques of Swedish Massage," on HolisticOnline .com, http://www.holistic-online.com/massage/mas_techniques .htm (accessed 6/12/06).

9. Ibid.

10. Richard Brennan, "What Is the Alexander Technique?" http://www.alexandertechnique.com/articles/brennan (accessed 6/12/06).

11. Ibid.

12. NCCAM Health Information: Acupuncture, http://nccam .nih.gov/health/acupuncture (accessed 6/12/06).

13. World Health Organization, WHO Fact Sheet Number 134, "Traditional Medicine," May 2003, http://www.who.int/

mediacentre/factsheets/fs134/en (accessed 6/12/06).

14. NCCAM Health Information: Whole Medical Systems: An Overview, http://nccam.nih.gov/health/backgrounds/wholemed .htm#nature (accessed 6/12/06).

15. Ibid., quoting M. J. Smith and A. C. Logan, "Naturopathy," *Medical Clinics of North America* 86(1) (2002): 173–184.

16. National Mental Health Information Center (U.S. Department of Health and Human Services, Substance Abuse and Mental Health Services Administration), FAQs, "Is treatment available for seasonal depression?" http://www.mentalhealth .samhsa.gov/highlights/december2004/sad/default.asp (accessed 6/12/06).

CHAPTER 8—MOTIVATION: KEEPING UP THE GOOD WORK

1. Joel Osteen, *Your Best Life Now: 7 Steps to Living at Your Full Potential* (New York: Warner Faith, 2004), 15.

2. Quoted in a number of sources, including http://www .albatrus.org/english/potpourri/quotes/martin_luther_quotes .htm; http://www.christiansquoting.org.uk/quote_w; http:// dailychristianquote.com/dcqluther.html.

3. Jack Canfield, Mark Victor Hansen, Les Hewitt, *The Power of Focus* (Deerfield Beach, FL: Health Communications, 2001).

4. Bill Johnson, *The Supernatural Power of a Transformed Mind* (Shippensburg, PA: Destiny Image, 2005), 114–15.

APPENDIX A: NUTRITION HELPS

1. Chestnut, *Innate Diet and Natural Hygiene.*

2. Ibid.

APPENDIX B: NATURAL REMEDIES GUIDE

1. Information in this charted adapted from Steven Bratman, MD, and David Kroll, PhD, *Natural Health Bible* (N.p.: Prima Lifestyles, 1999).

DIET

Balch, Phyllis A. *Prescription for Nutritional Healing: A Practical A-to-Z Reference to Drug-Free Remedies Using Vitamins, Minerals, Herbs and Food Supplements.* New York: Avery, 2000.

Colbert, Don, MD. *The Bible Cure for Weight Loss and Muscle Gain.* Lake Mary, FL: Siloam, 2000.

Gavin, William. *No White at Night: The Three Rule Diet.* New York: Riverhead, 2004.

Henner, Marilu, and Lorin Henner. *Healthy Kids: Help Them Eat Smart and Stay Active for Life.* New York: HarperCollins/ReganBooks, 2001.

Pratt, Steven G., and Kathy Matthews. *SuperFoods Rx: Fourteen Foods That Will Change Your Life.* New York: HarperCollins, 2003.

REST

Breedlove, Sally. *Choosing Rest: Cultivating a Sunday Heart in a Monday World.* Colorado Springs, CO: NavPress, 2002.

Dement, William C., and Christopher Vaughn. *The Promise of Sleep: A Pioneer in Sleep Medicine Explores the Vital Connection Between Health, Happiness, and a Good Night's Sleep.* New York: Random House/Dell, 2000.

Farrar, Steve, and Mary Farrar. *Overcoming Overload: Seven Ways to Find Rest in Your Chaotic World.* Sisters, OR: Multomah, 2003.

Muller, Wayne. *Sabbath: Restoring the Sacred Rhythm of Rest.* New York: Random House/Bantam, 1999.

Weissbluth, Marc. *Healthy Sleep Habits, Happy Child.* New York: Ballantine, 1999.

EXERCISE

Bailey, Covert. *Smart Exercise: Burning Fat, Getting Fit.* New York: Houghton-Mifflin, 1994.

Greene, Bob. *Get With the Program! Getting Real About Your Weight, Health, and Emotional Well-Being.* New York: Simon & Schuster, 2003.

Moffat, Marilyn, and Steve Vickery. *The American Physical Therapy Association Book of Body Maintenance and Repair.* New York: Henry Holt, 1999.

Phillips, Bill and Michael d-Orso. *Body for Life: 12 Weeks to Mental and Physical Strength.* New York: HarperCollins, 1999.

Waitz, Grete, and Gloria Averbuch. *On the Run: Exercise and Fitness for Busy People.* Emmaus, PA: Rodale, 1997.

ALTERNATIVE CARE

Castleman, Michael. *Nature's Cures: From Acupressure and Aromatherapy to Walking and Yoga, the Ultimate Guide to the Best Scientifically Proven, Drug-Free Healing Methods.* Emmaus, PA: Rodale, 1995.

Collinge, William. *The American Holistic Health Association Complete Guide to Alternative Medicine.* New York: Warner, 1996.

Pilzer, Paul Zane. *The Wellness Revolution.* New York: John Wiley & Sons, 2002.

Schuller, Robert A., and Douglas di Siena. *Possibility Living: Add*

Years to Your Life and Life to Your Years with God's Health Plan. New York: HarperCollins/HarperSanFrancisco, 2000.

International Chiropractors Association, Web site: http://www .chiropractic.org.

MOTIVATION

Carlson, Richard. *Don't Sweat the Small Stuff...and It's All Small Stuff.* New York: Hyperion, 1997.

Lerner, Ben. *Body by God.* Nashville: Thomas Nelson, 2003.

Peale, Norman Vincent. *The Power of Positive Thinking.* New York: Ballantine, 1996.

Siegel, Bernie. *Love, Medicine, and Miracles: Lessons Learned About Self-Healing From a Surgeon's Experience With Exceptional Patients.* New York: Harper, 1990.

More from DREAM Health

NOTE: No component of DREAM Health information is intended to diagnose, treat, or replace the advice of your health-care professional. I recommend that you consult your health-care professional before you take any product or engage in any DREAM Health protocol.

DREAMCOMPLETE

DREAMComplete *is a liquid vitamin and mineral supplement that can replenish the vital nutrition that has been lost in today's diet. DREAMComplete comes in liquid form and has been specially formulated from whole-food sea vegetation sources, so your body will absorb it naturally. DREAMComplete is 98 percent absorbable compared to pill form vitamins, which are only 10–20 percent absorbable.*

DREAMOMEGA

DREAMOmega *is a pure source of the omega-3 acids found in fish oil that have been proven to be vital to brain function, vascular conditioning, and overall optimal health. DREAMOmega replaces a significant deficiency of today's Western diet—with sufficiency.*

VISIT DREAMHEALTH.NET

Take your personal twenty-five-question health assessment and get your complete DREAM Health wellness plan at http://www .dreamhealth.net.

It's easy to order DREAM Health products. Visit the Web site at http://www.dreamhealth.net.

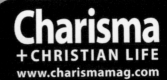